DEAD EXECS DON'T GET BONUSES

The Ultimate Guide to Surviving the C-Suite With a Healthy Heart

by Joel K. Kahn MD, FACC

Note to Readers

The information in this book should not be substituted for, or used to alter, medical therapy without your doctor's advice. For a specific health condition, see your physician for a consultation.

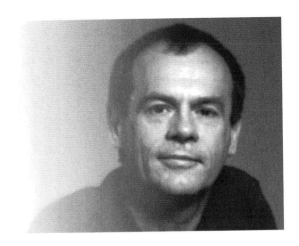

Imre Molnar
1951—2012

Dedication to Imre Molnar (1951-2012)

This book is dedicated to the memory of Imre Molnar, the Provost of the College for Creative Studies in Detroit, who died tragically of a heart attack in late 2012 while biking on vacation in California with his family. Under his leadership, the program in Detroit had grown to become one of the leading schools for automotive designers and he oversaw the graduation of many leading designers. His death was mourned worldwide for the loss of an extraordinary educator, family man and friend.

Acknowledgments

This book is the result of over a decade of medical training and 25 years of subsequent cardiology practice. Although there have been phenomenal advances in the treatment of heart disease in that time frame, we still have a long way to go. When the news headlines disclose the tragic loss of a highly productive person cut down in their prime by a heart attack - the number one killer in Western society - I am reminded that I cannot rest. Increasingly, my focus has been to educate as many people as possible on how to identify and reverse heart disease before it creates a tragic situation. I thank Joe Polish for the opportunity to present this topic to the Genius Network at the 25K Club meeting. The feedback was so strong that this book simply had to be written for wider distribution. I would also like to thank Mike Koenigs of Instant Customer for advancing my book writing and publishing skills. I'm grateful to all the teachers who helped me reach my current level of understanding of how to identify and prevent heart disease and reverse it if already established. Finally, I thank my wife Karen for always being supportive and understanding the long hours of practice and training that has gone into my formulation of this work.

Introduction: Heart Facts that Matter

Ron clearly did not look like he wanted anything to do with the appointment we had on Monday morning. He was dressed in an Italian suit and fine shoes and told me he was on his way to the airport to visit one of his manufacturing plants in South Carolina. I soon gleaned that he ran a large international corporation making electronic components for the automotive industry. When I asked why he was here, he answered: "My earlobes have a crease."

His wife had read an article I had written in Reader's Digest magazine as their Holistic Heart Doc columnist, where I described unusual clues to silent heart disease. I will come back to this and other signs of silent heart blockage later in the book; but regarding Ron, his wife had convinced him to get checked when she learned that my office was just a few miles from their home. He had just had a physical with his internist, had won the senior golf tournament at his club and prided himself on maintaining a trim waist as he approached 60. After discussing with him that heart disease can be silent for years before a heart attack or sudden death, and that his need for blood pressure cholesterol medication put him at increased risk, he agreed to further testing.

On his next appointment I reviewed with him imaging data of his heart and arteries which indicated that his arterial age was 10 years beyond his birth age, that he had asymptomatic heart disease and that he had a previously undiagnosed risk of artery damage, lipoprotein(a), which was eight times above normal. I spent time educating him about the importance of increased vegetables, fruits and whole grains and a reduction of processed meats, flours and sugars in his diet, as well as a number of supplements tailored to his individual risk profile (something called personalized lifestyle medicine).

In time, he clearly began to enjoy his visits. He enjoyed seeing the improvements in his advanced laboratory assessments and was relieved that we had found the disease early and that a plan to halt and reverse it was in place. When he asked me to do a webinar for his executives and key managers on heart disease detection and prevention, I was particularly pleased. This was because he was now not only my client but also my spokesperson, and I recently signed many copies of my book for him that he planned to give as holiday presents. To top it all off, the latest measurements of his artery functions have started to return toward normal for his age, something I am especially pleased about.

The statistics about the devastating effects of heart disease are easily accessible on the internet. A small amount of research will reveal that 600,000 people die of heart disease in the United States every year; one out of every four deaths in this country is due to cardiovascular diseases. Heart disease is a leading cause of death for both men and women - and causes far more deaths than cancer.

The particular type of heart disease I am focusing on in this book, coronary heart disease or a hardening of the arteries, kills nearly 400,000 people every year. One heart attack occurs roughly every 25 seconds and one person in this country dies as a result of heart disease or stroke around every 39 seconds. Every year, about 785,000 Americans have their first heart attack. The sheer scale of that number is mind-numbing. If one name, like Imre Molnar, can have such a profound personal impact on so many people, then multiply that by 785,000 and imagine all the pain and suffering that must be taking place and must end. I keep thinking of the University of Michigan Big House stadium, my alma mater, with a current capacity of just over 100,000 fans. Imagine filling that immense stadium every day for eight days with more than 100,000 moms, dads, sons, daughters, friends, co-workers... and every one of them suffers a heart attack, many fatal.

For another 470,000 people, a repeat heart attack occurs every year. That's enough to fill the Big House another fives times over with repeat heart events. Though those 470,000 have been in the Big House before, all of the resources of the medical community failed to prevent a recurrence. Finally, coronary heart disease is costing over $100 billion in the United States alone for health care services, medications and lost productivity.

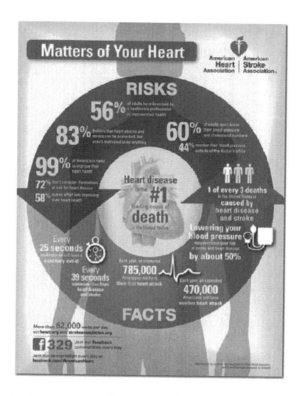

Figure 1. American Heart Association heart attack statistics

Although those statistics are daunting, we can learn more from single case studies. In a paper in the Stanford "Closer Look" series entitled Sudden Death of a CEO: Are Companies Prepared When Lightning Strikes? There is mention of the fact that seven CEOs of publicly-traded companies die suddenly each year, with heart attacks being the most common cause for the tragedy. When Jai Nagarkatti, CEO of Sigma-Aldrich, died suddenly due to a heart attack, business carried on as usual. A successor was named the very next day, thanks to a pre-existing succession plan. On the other hand, when Wendy's International CEO Gordon Teter died of a heart attack, his spot was not filled for months. Add to that the tragic deaths of Tim Russert and the actor James Gandolfini and it is clear that even high-profile persons capable of accessing the best medical care can lose their life at a young age. The list of CEOs dying from sudden heart attacks goes on and on: Kenneth Lay of Enron, Rick Lester of Target Research Group Arts, Jim Cantalupo of McDonald's, Ranjan Das of SAP, Paul McIlhenny of Tabasco, as well as many others, have died suddenly while running major businesses, leaving their families and their co-workers in distress.

The details of the careers and tragic deaths of these CEOs are a matter of public record and the disruption that followed their deaths was enormous. Take Ranjan Das for example. At age 42 he was the CEO of SAP for the Indian subcontinent region. He was the youngest CEO of a multinational corporation in India. He was returning home after using the corporate gym when he suffered a fatal cardiac arrest.

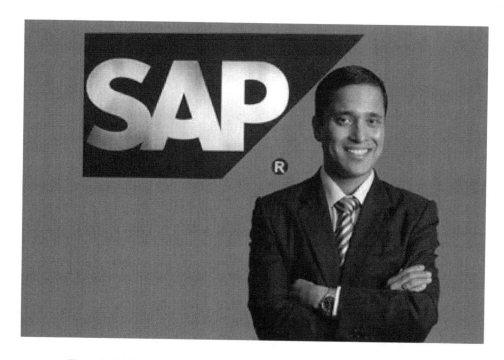

Figure 2. Ranjan Das, deceased CEO of SAP

Das was known for his healthy diet and exercise habits. He had finished a marathon months before his death (reminiscent of Jim Fixx, the world famous runner and author of The Complete Book of Running who died suddenly of heart disease at age 52). Das had led all marketing activities at SAP and designed and managed many revenue-generating functions involving software sales and support. He had previously founded a startup in Silicon Valley. He graduated MIT with a full scholarship and received an MBA from Harvard Business School. He wrote short stories and essays and was planning to make a movie. After his death, he left behind a wife and two children aged two and 10 years old. His tragic death is so enormous on so many levels. Whether or not advanced laboratory and imaging examinations (as are described later in this book) could have identified his silent heart disease, and whether lifestyle, supplemental, prescription drug and revascularization therapies could have been used to extend his life, will never be known... but we do not need any more stories like Ranjan Das. My sympathies go out to his family and friends.

James Cantalupo appeared to have it all. At age 60, he was the CEO of McDonalds. He was trained as an accountant and had a 30-year career with the food giant, starting as a controller, moving up to a regional manager, followed by head of the international business, then overall

CEO. Under his leadership he introduced salads, adult 'Happy Meals' and yogurt and fruit. He also served on the Board of Directors of Sears Roebuck Company. He was at a corporate convention in Orlando when he suddenly collapsed in his hotel room in the early morning hours, moments before he was due to speak to franchisees at the convention. He was rushed to a nearby hospital by ambulance with ongoing CPR but was pronounced dead on arrival, judged to have been killed by a fatal heart attack. He left a wife and two children. I can hardly imagine the shock, followed by the pain and suffering, that the family of Mr Cantalupo must have experienced, and my thoughts go out to them. I am certain that had he undergone the type of advanced evaluation outlined in this book, along with a treatment plan of lifestyle changes, supplements and periodic monitoring, his death could have been prevented.

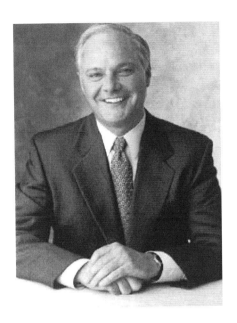

Figure 3. James Cantalupo, deceased CEO of McDonalds

On a further sad note, Cantalupo was replaced by 43-year-old

Charles Bell, the next COO and President of McDonalds. Within a year,

the Australian was diagnosed with colorectal cancer and died. Just before

his death, he was flown back to his native country to be amongst family

and friends when he took his last breath at such a tragically young age.

I was taught long ago that if you see people falling over a waterfall

into a deep body of water, a rapid response team is crucial to resuscitate them and save their lives. A higher goal, however, is to prevent people from falling over the waterfall in the first place. This analogy fits so well for the current status of the treatment of most coronary heart disease and heart attacks; we need to build a protective fence, so no one is catapulted over the falls into an uncertain future.

The goal of this book is to minimize the chances that you will suffer that fate. With all of the technological advances over the last few decades, it is possible to identify heart disease at a stage so early that treatment can be started years before a heart attack ever would have happened. Furthermore, simple lifestyle changes and certain medical treatments have been shown to prevent 90% of heart attacks, but such methods are rarely emphasized to executives in the C-suite. Finally, even established coronary heart disease and severely blocked arteries can be treated by diet and other modalities, resulting in a reversal of narrowing and an improvement in symptoms and outcome.

It is critical that more executives learn of these methods of living a heart attack-free life. I have invited a dear friend, Felicia Molnar, to share her story about the tragedy that struck her beloved husband Imre, cutting short his successful executive career in Detroit. I hope her words move you to action. Please, don't ignore the teachings in this book; share them with your friends, co-workers and family, and maximize the realistic goal of leaving a life free of heart disease and heart attacks.

"Bulletproof Your Heart" Summary:

1. One heart attack occurs every 35 seconds

2. Heart attacks are the leading cause of death in the Western world

3. Large companies have suffered the "lightning strike" of the death of a CEO

4. More than 90% of heart attacks are preventable

<u>ACTION STEP</u>

Read this book cover to cover and set up your advanced heart check-up ASAP so that lightning doesn't strike your C-suite.

As you can see, knowing facts about your heart matters.

To learn simple techniques which will help manage your day-to-day

stress from the comfort of your desk,

Visit www.drjoelkahn.com/deadexecs OR

Text **PREVENT** to 58885 OR

You can text your email address to 248-731-5145

On the website, you will find a video series that will walk you through stress management and breathing techniques you can easily implement into your busy schedule. You'll also find a PDF file to bring with you to your scheduled doctor appointment entitled, "Questions to Ask Your Doctor".

Chapter 1

Imre Molnar's Story (1951-2012) by Felicia Molnar

Those of us outside of the field of medicine have minds which are filled with stereotypes about the kind of person most likely to die from a heart attack. The guy who lives on French fries and a six-pack of beer is just one picture I can easily recall my husband conjuring up for himself; "That won't be me," he was thinking. He was a vegetarian, a swimmer and a cyclist. He quit drinking cold turkey in his late 30s and never touched another drop of alcohol. I assume that in his youth, he had indulged in the occasional joint and a cigarette or two; he was a product of the sixties after all. But by the time I met him, he was 40 years old and fighting fit. We were regularly bounding up mountains on our bicycles in California and Switzerland; free diving in the Red Sea and his native Australia; going to yoga classes in Bloomfield Hills. Imre was very athletic and to all who met him, he was a picture of health, strength, youthfulness and vitality. He held a senior executive position at an internationally-recognized school of art and design. He was provided with a generous salary and health care benefits. He travelled the world. He was the father of two relatively young children for his age.

For Imre, taking a break any day of the week involved some form of exercise. So on the morning of December 28th, 2012, while the rest of us were still sleepily recovering from Christmas Day celebrations, Imre announced plans to take a road ride with my cousin Jocelyn, herself a regular century rider. He promised our then 11-year-old son that they would be back from the ride in a couple of hours and that we would follow it up with a family hike up the Arroyo Trail to see the mountain sheep above the desert community of Borrego Springs, California, which lies 40 miles to the south of Palm Springs and at equal distance to San Diego. Borrego had become our regular early winter escape from Michigan with our Los Angeles-based friends and extended family. It was 75°F and sunny. I clearly remember the spring in his step as Imre pushed his beloved titanium-framed bicycle down the gravel driveway away from our vacation cottage. That was the last time we saw him alive.

About 50 minutes later I received a panicky call on Imre's phone from Jocelyn to come with the car and pick them up. Imre was not feeling well. She didn't sound normal but as I sped down the road in our rented Ford Crown Victoria, I was optimistic that perhaps he was just coming down with the stomach flu that had brought me and the kids to our knees on Boxing Day, after Christmas. I found them at mile marker 16 and as I pulled up, a California Highway Patrol Officer was already on the scene. Jocelyn was performing CPR and the officer had his trunk open and his paddles out. Soon an ambulance from the Borrego Springs Fire Department arrived and for the next two hours, four medics worked to bring my beloved husband of 20 years back to life. They tore off his cycling jersey and shoes. There were doctors on the radios, and there were even a few moments when they got a heartbeat and considered calling in a helicopter. I kept away, pacing among the cactus and saying my yoga mantra - Om Namah Shivaya - over and over again. It was the only prayer I knew. But finally, all of the work stopped and Imre was pronounced dead by a doctor who had even never set eyes on him before. Spontaneously, I lay down with him on the side of that road for more than an hour, shivering as the sun went down, contemplating the horror of letting him go. My mind raced with the shock of what lay before me, including the blackest thought of all: our children, fatherless and heartbroken. While I held on to his lifeless body, the medics and first responders kept me safe from the traffic speeding by on the highway. Eventually, a sweet fireman convinced me to return back to the house where our two children, our 18-year-old Japanese exchange student, my mother and our friends had already received the shocking news. I was informed that the coroner's office would be delayed in retrieving the body; an autopsy was required by the County of San Diego Medical Examiner because he had died outside of a hospital. I myself had no idea what had killed him, and though it pained me to know that his body would be in limbo and alone in the County morgue of all places, I was desperate for some explanation to give meaning to his inconceivable death. On New Year's Eve, the doctor from the Coroner's office finally called with the results and the cause of death.

In no uncertain terms he told me that Imre had had pervasive heart disease and had died from a massive blow to his lower anterior artery, or, the "Widow Maker", as it is profoundly better known. I was in further shock.

A month later, I had resigned my job and a memorial was held at the college where more than 1,000 people turned out to honor Imre's work and life. It took nearly a year for the college to name his successor. On the financial front, I was busy with lawyers and investment advisors who took me under their wings to forge the way forward, which was a terrifying prospect. Luckily, we were (and still are) well-provided for, thanks to the financial stewardship we had put in place including wills, life insurance policies, social security for the children and some angels who offered work, which provided me with the ability to keep our ship afloat. I am grateful on all scores for the people who stepped forward to help and the fact that our financial house was in order. This forward planning allowed me and the children to proceed with our emotional healing without the stress of not knowing where our next meal would come from or how we would pay our bills.

Dead Execs Don't Get Bonuses

To be perfectly honest, there were some developing but subtle signs of Imre's possible heart disease, including compromised breathing in the form of a nagging cough that came and went with the seasons. However, his regular internist, a friend, had conducted pulmonary tests and convinced him that a virus was causing the congestion. The doctor prescribed a teaspoon of codeine-laced cough syrup nightly to deal with the annoyance, but I don't think Imre had ever touched the Costco-sized bottle. Imre also had slightly elevated cholesterol, but he was told by his two family doctors that it did not require medication or any further intervention. Imre was busy running a huge and ever-increasing multi-million dollar institution and doctors' appointments were always seen as an inconvenience. He never pressed on for any further tests. He was a 60-year-old grown man and quite frankly, I didn't marry him to be a nagging mother-figure in his life.

I am here to tell you - as Imre is not - that your mind will thwart and delude you about such matters as your own health and even the health of those that you love. It may not come as a surprise, but our own survival is not necessarily guaranteed by our egocentric mind, which we all selfishly assume will be our number one protector. I truly believe that the failure to deeply know our own health rests in our own lack of self-education about the very silent and pernicious killer that is heart disease. You hold in your hand the remedy. You are already ahead of the game, just by reading this book.

It is my own personal mission to see the end of heart disease. I want to be one of the last people standing here in a spot which you never want to find yourself standing in: having joined the lonely club of widows whose partners have passed way before their prime, leaving young children and spouses to prematurely fend for themselves. But sadly, people are still dying every day from heart disease, leaving families in shock, children bereft and colleagues and institutions backpedalling to recover their missions after facing the traumatic, unexpected loss of their leader. This is a disease that Dr. Kahn and I believe is preventable and even, dare I posit, extinguishable. But first, you must educate yourself, embrace your intuition and dare to challenge your health care providers with proactive questions which will demand even more inquiry. The old adage that "No

one will save you if you don't know how to save yourself" works well

here. You certainly know your health and your body's capabilities better

than anyone. You know best when you feel that your activity is

compromised. Don't blame lowering activity levels on age only. Dig

deeper. When a cough lingers well beyond the course of a normal cold, be

suspicious. When you get off your bike and start experiencing shortness of

breath, be curious - even if you only eat three meals of green vegetables

and only ever once put your lips around the filter of a cigarette. Normality

does change with age, but lingering coughs, shortness of breath, creases in

your earlobe, digestive issues and other more obvious signs, like high

blood pressure and cholesterol, demand that you pay attention and track

down a cause. Heart disease wants you to miss the signs, it wants to win;

but you can outsmart it.

Today, two years since the passing of my husband, I walk around

with a lot of questions of "what if". I repeatedly berate myself for my lack

of action on behalf of my soulmate's health. My lack of action was clearly inadvertent and unintentional; his best interests were always in my heart, thoughts and actions, even if he never made the bed or mostly left the toilet seat up. There is no way to undo the damage; now, it is simply too late. Posthumously, I am aware of all the signs I missed that I simply did not know I was missing. I believe I have a responsibility to humanity to attempt to educate people to avoid repeating my errors, and it is my personal quest to try and prevent the suffering which my children and I carry around with us daily. I am in the process of forgiving myself; of recognizing that the number one lesson here is that I should have trusted my intuition and dragged my reluctant husband off to a specialist after his intern told him more than twice that his lungs were just fine and it was probably a pesky virus that was causing his exercised-induced asthma. I can't afford to beat myself up about this any longer, but this healing comes with a promise of action: to work on my mission together with Dr. Kahn to end heart disease. Please join us!

ACTION STEP

It's clear Felicia always had Imre's best interests at heart; however, the inadvertent lack of action to ensure that his heart was healthy is something that was life-changing for the entire family! As you can see, knowing facts about your heart matters.

To learn simple techniques which will help manage your day-to-day

stress from the comfort of your desk,

Visit www.drjoelkahn.com/deadexecs OR

Text **PREVENT** to 58885 OR

You can text your email address to 248-731-5145

On the website, you will find a video series that will walk you through

stress management and breathing techniques you can easily implement

into your busy schedule. You'll also find a PDF file to bring with you to

your scheduled doctor appointment entitled, "Questions to Ask Your

Doctor".

Chapter 2

Coronary Heart Disease: Just the Facts

"Remembering that you are going to die is the best way I know to avoid

the trap of thinking you have something to lose."

Steve Jobs, CEO of Apple

Dave was lucky, because he had a wife who was worried about his stress levels and the long hours he put into running the family automotive manufacturing business. Jane had read an article that I had written for Reader's Digest magazine on unusual signs of silent heart disease. In it, I mentioned that erectile dysfunction or sexual difficulties can be the first sign in men that arteries are being attacked by damaging factors. Although

Dave was not eager to discuss it, his ability to achieve and maintain an erection was far less reliable in his 50s than a decade earlier, and Jane showed him my article. He reluctantly came in to see me, though he would not tell anyone at the check-in window why he had made the appointment. He stubbornly told me: "My wife made me come in," and it wasn't until we almost parted that he indicated his issue was a bedroom check-up. As I outline in this book, he underwent a "CARE-full" evaluation of the status of his arteries, lifestyle and biochemistry and he was found to have silent heart artery - and likely penal artery - disease, due to atherosclerosis. As I often tell my male patients, being hard is a pleasure... except when it describes your arteries. With time, I was able to break down his resistance to recognizing that his diet, exercise program (or lack thereof), sleep patterns, late-night snacking and growing waistline were all factors which put him at risk of a fatal heart attack, while already manifesting themselves as sexual dysfunction. A year later, he had dropped 18 pounds of weight and his waist was no longer 42 but 36 inches; he was making exercise a priority, he had added five servings of vegetables to his daily program (using morning green smoothies to start the day), and was sleeping seven hours at night with some natural supplements and meditation. Oh, and by the way, his bedroom antics were back to a more youthful level, making him and Jane smile on visits.

Generally, we are all born with three coronary arteries which continuously feed blood to our hearts. They are called the coronary arteries because they form a corona, or crown, around the heart. They are approximately three to four millimeters in diameter and taper as they give off branches. As the heart pumps freshly oxygenated blood around the body, the first thing it does is to feed these coronary arteries so that they can maintain its life-sustaining function. Coronary heart disease has existed for generations and has even been found in Egyptian mummies, as determined by CAT scan images of their arteries. Eskimos living in isolated areas of the world have been found to have this same disease, perhaps due to their ultra-high fat blubber diet. There are certain societies, however, which have traditionally been almost 100% free of this killer, such as Uganda and Papua New Guinea; much has been learned by studying their lifestyles. Although at first, coronary heart disease was felt to be an unavoidable byproduct of aging, the Framingham Heart Study in Framingham, Massachusetts (initially published in 1961), demonstrated that certain characteristics predispose individuals to progressive narrowing and blockage of the heart arteries. This process is often called coronary artery disease. The Framingham study determined that smoking, diabetes mellitus, high blood pressure, high cholesterol and having a first-degree relative with early heart disease predicted early narrowing of heart arteries. Furthermore, studies in the 1970s demonstrated that certain individuals have a genetic defect in their cholesterol metabolism. About one person in every 400 inherits a bad gene from their parents which raises their cholesterol levels significantly and causes heart disease decades earlier than most. One person in a million receives two bad cholesterol genes (one from each parent) and as a result, heart disease can develop fatally - even in teenagers. I myself personally cared for an 11-year-old girl who required bypass surgery due to this condition. These children teach us how important blood cholesterol is in forming heart disease.

Coronary heart disease can develop progressively and most often proceeds without any symptoms. It has been found in people as young as 19 and 20 years old. Soldiers in the Korean War who died during battle had autopsies which often showed early signs of coronary artery disease; this has also been found in soldiers who died during the Vietnam and Iraq wars. Slowly and progressively, the arteries narrow without any outward signs or symptoms. Generally, cardiologists observe that an artery has to have been narrowed by more than 70% to have the potential to rob the heart of sufficient blood during activity that it brings on warning symptoms during exertion. The classic symptom is called angina pectoris, from the Latin for "choking in the chest". This description goes back several hundred years. The classic scenario features an individual who, shortly after a meal, exerts themselves in cold weather and subsequently develops a pressure, tightness or squeezing in the central chest area and possibly into the neck or arms. By stopping and resting, these symptoms go away within a couple of minutes. However, by the time these symptoms have manifested themselves, the process has been progressing

for years undetected. There are other symptoms of advanced blockages,

including jaw pain, back pain, sweating, nausea, a racing heart, fatigue,

ear or head pain and shortness of breath. These may be the symptoms

found more commonly in women with clogged arteries. Again, by the time

these symptoms develop, at least one and often multiple arteries have very

advanced disease.

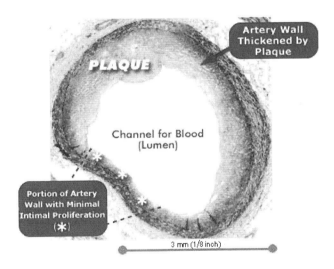

Figure 4. Silent plaque narrowing a heart artery in a young person

This is the reason that for many patients, once the first time

symptoms of coronary heart disease have presented themselves, the next step is a bypass operation or a stent, because the disease is so advanced. How can this process, which kills more people than any other disease in the Western world, go undetected for so many years? How can people have had complete examinations from their health care provider, often including some heart testing, yet walk out of the office and still have an undetected and advanced heart condition? How did President Bill Clinton have so many advanced medical examinations during his presidency and still present with advanced heart disease requiring bypass surgery just a couple years later? This will be talked about in detail in future chapters.

There are some other clues to coronary heart disease that are important to recognize. In men, erectile dysfunction, or problems achieving and maintaining an erection, have been studied and can predict the presence of coronary heart disease. Of course, there are clearly physical and psychological reasons for erectile dysfunction which have nothing to do with the heart. However, the mechanism of an erection, requiring healthy arteries which can accommodate a major increase in blood flow on demand, is driven by the same factors which determine whether heart arteries are healthy or not. Smoking, elevated blood pressure and blood sugar, elevated cholesterol, excessive weight, inactivity, poor dietary choices and other factors which can be measured will damage arteries throughout the body. Scientific bodies have recommended that men with erectile dysfunction have an evaluation of their risk for heart disease. In my clinic, this includes a very thorough and accurate determination of the health of the heart arteries.

Another clue to coronary heart disease involves the leg arteries. One symptom, called intermittent claudication, manifests itself in the form of cramping in the thighs or calves during or immediately after exertion. This is the equivalent to the angina that occurs in the chest, but is the result of arteries in the legs being severely or completely blocked. This is most common in smokers, but can occur in other settings, as well. If there is a feeling of cramping of the calves or thighs while walking, not only do the legs need to be evaluated, but the heart must be, as well. The wry joke is that the reason the Marlboro man was always riding a horse was that his legs were so clogged up he couldn't walk.

Dead Execs Don't Get Bonuses

Another unusual sign of possible silent coronary heart disease takes us all the way up to the earlobe. Over the last several decades, reports have suggested that a diagonal deep crease in the earlobe is predictive of silent coronary heart disease, though no one knows exactly why. I learned of this strange association long ago in medical school, but it seemed to have fallen out of favor for a while. More recently, advanced imaging techniques of the heart have demonstrated that it is actually of high predictive value. It's worth taking a look at your own earlobe - if there's a deep crevice in the lower part of the ear, an evaluation of your overall risk of heart disease and an advanced imaging session may be worthwhile.

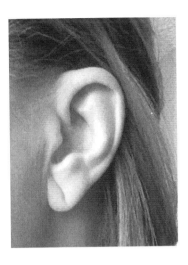

Figure 5. A picture of an earlobe crease as a sign of silent heart disease

Another potential clue to silent heart disease involves your sleeping habits. With every passing year, more and more people are becoming overweight and obese. Sleep disturbances, including sleep apnea, are rising in frequency - primarily because obesity is one of the causes. Snoring excessively and periodically stopping breathing during sleep is very common. It doesn't only occur, however, in overweight people. A high frequency of silent coronary heart disease is found in individuals with sleep apnea symptoms, as confirmed by appropriate sleep apnea testing.

Baldness, particularly at the top of the head, has been shown to correlate with early heart disease. The exact mechanism is not clear; however, it should prompt consideration for testing for silent heart disease.

Although there are classic symptoms and less common warning signs, my recommendation is that every executive get an advanced screening for silent coronary heart disease to avoid a tragic or fatal heart attack. Too often, the first symptom of coronary heart disease is a cardiac arrest and death; this book describes a system to dramatically decrease the chances of that ever happening. Let's move on to discussing how doctors usually identify blocked heart arteries and how more advanced imaging techniques (which have been available for years) can dramatically improve this process.

"Bulletproof Your Heart" Summary

1. Heart disease slowly progresses and is silent for years, but is rarely detected

2. Angina is a chest pressure or shortness of breath on exertion

3. Sexual dysfunction, baldness, leg pain and earlobe creases are early clues

4. The first symptom of heart disease is often sudden death - a bad deal.

ACTION STEP

If you suffer exertional angina chest discomfort or intermittent claudication you should seek out a cardiologist and be seen right away. If you have sleep disturbances, erectile dysfunction, a deep earlobe crease or premature baldness, keep on reading this book and set up a plan to be checked.

Now that you have the facts, you might want to take the next step. To learn simple techniques which will help manage your day-to-day stress from the comfort of your desk,

Visit www.drjoelkahn.com/deadexecs OR

Text **PREVENT** to 58885 OR

You can text your email address to 248-731-5145

On the website, you will find a video series that will walk you through stress management and breathing techniques you can easily implement into your busy schedule. You'll also find a PDF file to bring with you to your scheduled doctor appointment entitled, "Questions to Ask Your Doctor".

Chapter 3

Does a Check-Up Check Anything?

"It's in our best interests to put some of the old rules aside

and create new ones."

Robert Iger, CEO of Walt Disney

Meredith looked stunned when I met her on a stretcher in the emergency room of my local hospital. My pager had indicated that an urgent consultation for chest pain was requested. She was still dressed in her street clothes, although she was on a stretcher in a gown, with oxygen in her nose and an IV in her hand. Multiple IV medications were infusing into her veins, including nitroglycerin and a blood-thinner called heparin.

She kept shaking her head and looking at her cell phone. She told me she had an important meeting in the morning and as it was 4pm in the afternoon, she wanted to know what the plan was. I asked her questions, examined her through her clothes and reviewed the data available in the emergency room. She was 59 years old and ran a large non-profit organization dedicated to cancer prevention. She had a long history of business leadership positions during her career and was well known in the community. When I asked her about exercise, she snorted, indicating that her job, her home commitments and her aging parents had interrupted her pilates exercises long ago. She was often traveling in an airplane to meet donors, eating on the run, sleeping in uncomfortable hotels and had gained 22 pounds in the last five years since menopause. When I reviewed her laboratory results and electrocardiogram, it was apparent that she had suffered a small heart attack, most likely from a severely blocked heart artery. When I told her my assessment, she gave me a rather cold look and said: "Impossible." Indeed, she had just had a "complete" physical exam two months earlier and was told that the results were excellent. And now this? I was able to arrange a cardiac catheterization within two hours, identify a nearly completely blocked heart artery to the back of her heart and place a drug-coated stent to resolve the blockage. She was able to be discharged the next day before lunch, but had to reschedule her important meeting. In subsequent visits, we explored how her lifestyle habits had slipped to the point where she had developed nearly fatal heart disease and how a routine physical examination can miss finding this problem at an early stage. Fortunately, she is now 18 months on from this scary day and has changed priorities in her life to make time for good sleep, excellent nutrition and fitness classes five days a week. She has put her administrative skills to good use, deciding to administer her own health.

Why aren't more heart attacks prevented? Why isn't early heart disease diagnosed more frequently in the current medical model? Although it is widely recognized that heart disease is a serious problem and the leading cause of death in the Western world, the current medical model simply doesn't recognize that there are techniques available for early diagnosis, early identification of underlying causes and early preventive strategies. A physical exam around the age of 50 will almost always include a recommendation for a colonoscopy. Colorectal cancer is a serious medical illness that must be identified early. How do we go about doing this? We pass a scope through the rectum and the entire colon, looking directly at this target organ for early signs of precancerous or cancerous lesions. A woman around the age of 50 will be recommended to have a mammogram or some other form of direct breast imaging. Breast cancer clearly is a serious disorder. The mammogram or other breast imaging approaches directly image the breast, attempting to find evidence of lesions at the earliest stages.

But what about the heart? What do most people receive when visiting their doctor at the age of 40 or 50? Usually, the examination will include measurements of weight, waist size, blood pressure and laboratory values including a cholesterol panel and fasting blood sugar. Sometimes an electrocardiogram (ECG with a C for cardiac or EKG with a K for Kardiac from the Dutch) is performed, but the administrative panels which make recommendations about the contents of a physical exam usually omit even the simple ECG. Questions about smoking and questions about family history of heart disease are obtained. If desired, that basic panel of information can be plugged into a Framingham Risk Score calculator which you can find online and which can give a prediction of the risk of heart disease events like a heart attack or death over the next 10 years. In my experience, this is done in well under 10% of most physical exams. Even if it is calculated, it still begs for personalized accuracy, since it is simply a general calculation from a group of persons in Massachusetts who may be quite different from your profile.

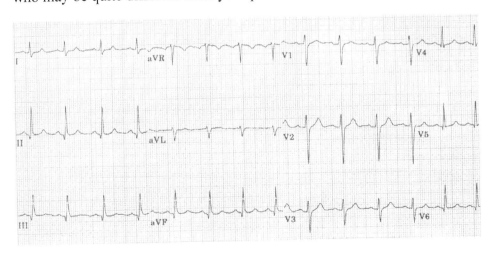

Figure 6. A normal ECG in a patient with advanced heart

blockages

What about ways of identifying silent heart disease that a doctor might consider in today's practice? For years, the concept of an executive physical stress test has been promoted. Actually, it hasn't been promoted or recommended by the American College of Cardiology; doctors have simply struggled to find something more than their stethoscope to give some insight into the state of the heart. In fact, the American College of Cardiology recommends against stress testing in asymptomatic persons without known heart disease. Why? The answer is that there are so many inaccurate predictions which come from stress testing in this group that the result is a huge amount of anxiety and additional and potentially harmful and unnecessary procedures. How can this be?

I have been involved in exercise stress testing, including nuclear cardiology testing, for 30 years. I have personally interpreted over 100,000 exercise stress tests. I wrote one of the first research papers in the world on using the agent Cardiolite for imaging of the heart, now the most frequently-used nuclear agent there is. My experience has shown that even the most sophisticated of exercise stress tests, the nuclear stress test using Cardiolite or Myoview, has great inaccuracies. Studies show that if your heart arteries are narrowed at least 70% or more by coronary artery disease, the chances are 70% that a routine exercise treadmill stress test will show an abnormality which identifies silent heart disease. That means that 30% of the time, this advanced heart artery lesion is missed. Furthermore, if the heart artery lesion is 40% to 60% narrowed, for example, it's almost certainly going to be missed and a normal result will give reassurance that no heart disease is present when that is grossly wrong.

If you change the type of exercise stress test to a stress echocardiogram or stress nuclear study using Myoview or Cardiolite, the numbers may reach 85% accuracy in detecting a heart artery lesion that has narrowed by 70% or more. However, that still means that 15% of people walking away from a stress test which was read as normal actually have advanced heart artery disease. The opposite side of the coin is also true. Using a routine exercise treadmill test, 20% to 30% of patients with completely normal (or only mildly diseased heart arteries) will be flagged as showing abnormal results, indicative of coronary artery disease. This person will be informed of the abnormality, leading to increased stress and anxiety over the concern of a diagnosis of silent heart disease. It is very likely that medical treatment and further testing (which might even include an invasive cardiac authorization) will be recommended. No matter who performs an invasive cardiac catheterization, there is always risk of bleeding, allergies to medications and even death. I have performed over 10,000 of these procedures and am well aware of the potential risks.

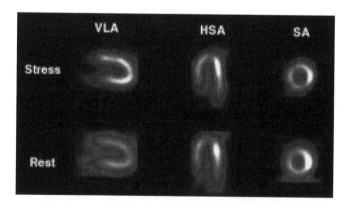

Figure 7. A normal nuclear heart scan in a patient with 50% heart blockages

If the more sophisticated stress echocardiogram or stress nuclear exercise test is performed, still around 15% of people with normal heart arteries will show some abnormality on the study; and again, further treatment and testing is likely. This is all such a mess in asymptomatic persons that medical bodies like the American College of Cardiology do not recommend a routine exercise stress test for screening for silent heart. Exceptions can include patients with high risk jobs, such as airline pilots, and patients with multiple risk factors, such as patients with diabetes who smoke, simply because their initial risk of heart disease is so high before the test. I hope you agree with me that the current practices for the detection of silent heart artery disease - the number one killer in the Western world (including the number one killer of executives) - leave much to be desired and improved upon.

"Bulletproof Your Heart Summary"

1. Standard physical examinations are inadequate to detect silent heart disease

2. Stress tests are not recommended as screening tests

3. Stress tests are fraught with false readings

4. Stress tests can only identify advanced heart disease

ACTION STEP

If your doctor recommends a screening stress test, particularly if it is a nuclear stress test exposing you to high radiation counts, discuss the accuracy with your healthcare provider. Routine and metabolic stress tests are available at higher end health clubs and can measure your fitness with less risk and adequate information.

Now that we have explored routine checkups, be sure to take advantage

of the bonus techniques which will help manage your day-to-day stress

from the comfort of your desk

Visit www.drjoelkahn.com/deadexecs OR

Text **PREVENT** to 58885 OR

You can text your email address to 248-731-5145

On the website, you will find a video series that will walk you through

stress management and breathing techniques you can easily implement

into your busy schedule. You'll also find a PDF file to bring with you to

your scheduled doctor appointment entitled, "Questions to Ask Your

Doctor".

Chapter 4

Coronary Calcium CT Scans: Know Your Score Now

"The common question that gets asked in business is: 'Why?' That's a good question, but an equally valid question is, 'Why not?'"

Jeff Bezos, CEO of Amazon

Terry counted his blessings on a daily basis. Great children, a great wife and a great real estate business. He watched his children assume more responsibility, allowing him more time in his late 60s to slow down a bit; it was about that time that he heard about CT scans for screening for silent diseases, including heart disease and cancer. As a center had just opened up nearby, he figured it couldn't hurt to get checked - retirement years were now close at hand and he didn't want to miss out on the good life. He had no symptoms of heart issues, he was thin and he passed all of his doctor visits, so he was confident the results would be reassuring. When he got a message at work to call the imaging center, he was prepared for great news. In fact, he was told that his coronary arteries were heavily calcified in the most serious sections, with a total score well over 1,000, and it was important that he see a heart specialist. For a while, he thought it was a joke planned by one of his friends - but when he checked the number on the phone, he knew it was no joke. Within two weeks he had a stress test with imaging pictures. The report indicated poor blood flow to the front of his heart, even though he had no chest tightness or pressure when on the treadmill. After careful consideration of the risks, he had a cardiac catheterization (angiogram) showing a severe narrowing of his left main heart artery (LMCA) and within an hour, a cardiac surgeon was at his bedside discussing bypass surgery to his heart. He could not believe the sequence of events, but after listening to the pro and cons, he decided to schedule an elective heart operation. Fortunately it was uncomplicated and three new bypasses were placed to his blocked heart arteries. He went home four days later and was back in the office in a mere six weeks.

It's time for the good news. There is no way you can have read the prior chapter and come away feeling good about the fact that most executive physical exams have no chance of picking up even advanced silent heart artery disease, let alone earlier cases. About 20 years ago, advances in technology reached the arena of computed tomography scans, or CT scans. CT scans were an amazing breakthrough in the 1970s, but the initial devices had single imaging elements and were quite slow in their acquisition of data. A breakthrough came when a small company called Imatron developed a new approach to CT scanning. This was called electron beam CT scanning, or EBCT. These machines started to be mass-produced and sold in the 1990s and were many times faster than the traditional CT scanner. CT scanning of the heart prior to this time was not practical because the heart was always in motion and CT scans on early generation standard machines produced very blurry images. However, the

EBCT machine was able to provide a scan of sufficient speed to identify portions of the heart accurately. Even though no contrast dye was injected, the arteries which feed the heart with blood could be seen because they travel surrounded by a bed of fat. The arteries are filled with liquid blood that has a different density than fat; therefore, the arteries could be imaged through several generation branches quite easily with these new machines in a matter of seconds.

My apologies for the digression, but I must provide some background on why all of this matters for early heart disease detection in patients without classic symptoms. For nearly 100 years since X-ray imaging began to be applied in a variety of medical situations, it was noticed that calcium deposits, similar to what was seen on X-rays over bony areas like ribs, could be seen in what appeared to be the distribution of arteries. For example, an X-ray of the leg taken because of a fracture was capable of showing calcification that seemed to course along with the arteries of the leg in a diabetic patient. Similarly, calcification on a chest X-ray in portions which correlated with the aorta, the body's largest blood vessel, could be identified - even though the purpose of the chest X-ray might have been quite different, such as evaluating a cough, for example. Therefore, calcification of arteries as an abnormal discovery of X-rays was quite well-known when the EBCT machine was introduced. Furthermore, both basic and human research had shown that calcification was a marker of atherosclerosis or hardening of the arteries. In almost every situation where plaque develops in an artery and leads to progressive narrowing, calcification is a portion of the elements, often contributing up to 20% of the volume of the plaque. The density of a calcified artery is very different than the density of the blood within the artery or the density of the fat around the artery. The bottom line is that it's very easy to detect calcium in an artery. Therefore, it's actually very easy to detect plaque in an artery, using calcium as the marker of the plaque. However, until the EBCT approach became available, this wasn't true in heart arteries in an accurate manner. All of that changed with the EBCT scanner.

Much of the credit for the utilization of the EBCT scanner in protecting silent calcified heart arteries goes to Dr. Arthur Agatston, who is still practicing as a cardiologist in the Miami area. He recognized that the new scanner could detect silent heart artery disease and was involved in developing a software program which measured how much calcium was present over the heart arteries. He developed a score, often called the Agatston Score, indicating levels of calcium in the arteries. He saw that some results of the EBCT scan of the heart had a calcium score of zero, because no calcium was detected in any artery. Meanwhile, he also saw that some people had calcium deposits in heart arteries which were so heavy that the score could be in the hundreds or even thousands. This opened a whole new era of heart artery detection in patients without symptoms. Dr. Agatston never patented the software and scoring method, but we do not need to feel too badly about that; he went on to write the South Beach diet books and has done quite well for himself.

The EBCT scanners were very expensive and the centers that started to offer the scans were charging hundreds and hundreds of dollars, which were not covered by insurance. Still, many people in the 1990s paid these dollars for the scans, just like Terry, whose story started this chapter.

Nevertheless, the high cost and exclusive nature of the EBCT machine meant that most people did not have access to this groundbreaking new technology.

Manufacturers like General Electric and other producers of standard CT scanners reacted. They developed faster scanners which were called multi-slice; these are the kind of CT scanners that are still used in practice today. Although there was quite a controversy over whether the EBCT or the multi-slice scans were of equal accuracy, ultimately the multi-slice CT scanners became the market leader. They could be used for many other body imaging purposes and on the whole, they were just more practical. They were also more widely available. GE bought Imatron as it was fading and nowadays, EBCT is no longer available. Over time, the price of the multi-slice CT scan gradually began to drop. Even today, most health insurance plans will not cover this cardiac examination; but fortunately, the price has dropped to the range of $200 or less. In my community, several centers offer the coronary artery calcium scans for under $100.

What can you expect from having a coronary artery calcium scan? I had one done to check my heart arteries at age 50 and am proud to say my score was zero. The test does not involve the need for an IV or the injection of any medication. I simply laid down on the table and was pushed into the CT scanner. I held my breath a couple of times for about 10 seconds and the entire examination was done in under a minute. It was not claustrophobic. Nobody can be allergic because there is no medication given. Also, even persons with a pacemaker or other metal devices are capable of having the scan. The only limitation might be a weight limitation, as many CT scanners are limited in patients over 350 to 400 pounds.

Who should not have the coronary calcium scan? If someone already knows they have coronary artery disease, perhaps after a previous cardiac catheterization has shown blockage, after a previous heart stent or after a previous heart bypass surgery, there would be no need for a screening test of this type. People who know that they have blockage in other parts of the body, such as an artery of the brain called the carotid artery or the arteries of the leg, remain debatable candidates for the CT

scan. These people are going to need treatment with modalities like aspirin

and lifestyle medicine, regardless of what is found in the heart. However,

in my practice, I find that if I can tell a patient that the disease also

involves the heart arteries, putting them at risk for the number one killer in

the Western world, they get even more motivated to adhere to a prevention

and reversal lifestyle. The American College of Cardiology has given a

high endorsement to the use of coronary artery calcium scans in persons

with known risk factors for silent coronary disease - those risk factors we

discussed in the previous chapter. In my view, however, risk factors are

only partially able to risk-stratify a person accurately; I personally discuss

a coronary calcium scan to identify silent heart disease even in persons

without obvious risk factors.

What about risks of the CT scan? Other than the cost, the only

other concerns would be radiation, the possibility of creating undue stress

and soft plaque.

Let's talk about radiation. For decades, cardiologists have relied on exercise nuclear testing using treadmill examinations, as was discussed in the previous chapter. Although we were always aware of the radiation risks to the patient, there were not many alternatives and there wasn't much discussion of this risk. One measure of the dose of radiation is called a millisievert or mSv. An exercise test with Cardiolite may expose a patient to roughly 12 to 15 mSv of radiation. By comparison, a cardiac catheterization done in an efficient manner may expose a patient to about 10 mSv of radiation. What about coronary artery calcium CT scans? In centers with the most advanced multi-slice scanners, which now are often 64 slice, 128 slice, 256 slice and beyond, the imaging has gotten so fast that the radiation dose may be only 1 mSv or less. The amount of radiation is so much less for calcium CT scans (compared with the popular exercise nuclear stress test) and the information obtained is so much more accurate that I favor the CT scan. Finally, there is a multivitamin/antioxidant packet that can be taken 45 minutes before the CT scan and has been shown to reduce potential DNA damage from imaging radiation (Bioshield R1, Premier Micronutrients Inc.). I recommend this for all tests which involve radiation exposure.

The other limitations of calcium CT scans include the fact that people given a zero score could take it to mean that they can live it up and forget about preventive strategies, though in my experience, this has not happened. On the other hand, persons with mildly abnormal scans could get unduly anxious about the heart disease diagnosis. Again, I have not seen this often, largely because I offer them so many preventive options. Finally, some plaques do not contain enough calcium to be detected, so-called "soft plaques". These can evade detection and are a concern in patients with angina, such as those seen in the emergency room. However, for those without any suspicious symptoms going for elective scheduled outpatient coronary calcium CT scans, this has not proven to be an important limitation.

An allergy to iodine or shellfish is not a reason to avoid one of these scans. As no contrast agents are used and nothing is injected (not even an IV is started), there is no concern about allergic reactions (as opposed to contrast CT scans such as coronary CT angiography, which can provoke life-threatening allergic responses).

What have we learned?

Simply put, your coronary artery calcium score may be the most important test in saving your life. For example, the European Society of cardiology developed a positional statement about cardiac CT scans. Their statement was: "There is overwhelming evidence that coronary calcification represents a strong marker of risk for future cardiovascular events in asymptomatic individuals and has prognostic power above and beyond traditional risk factors". The same positional statement indicated that in asymptomatic individuals, a calcium score of zero was associated with a very low risk of heart events over the next three to five years (less than 1% per year). Individuals with a coronary calcium score greater than 1,000 have an 11-fold increase in risk of major events, even if they are without symptoms. This is a huge difference.

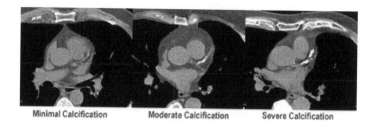

Minimal Calcification Moderate Calcification Severe Calcification

Figure 8. Examples of mild, moderate and severe heart artery calcification showing as white in the middle of the heart, shadowed in grey

The Texas Heart Institute summarized the evidence for coronary calcium scoring. They indicated that using standard risk factors such as cholesterol and blood pressure, at least 25% of people with heart artery disease are completely missed. They felt that coronary artery calcium scoring was important because "the presence of coronary artery calcium indicates underlying coronary heart disease with essentially NO false positive findings." They also went on to say that "a calcium score of zero in asymptomatic low risk adults makes the presence of atherosclerotic plaque or significant luminal obstructive disease highly unlikely and is associated with a very low risk of cardiovascular events within two to five years. Conversely, positive coronary calcium scores confirmed the presence of coronary atherosclerotic plaque and rising scores are directly proportional to the increased coronary heart disease risk. In particular, coronary calcium scores higher than 100 are associated with a high risk greater than 2% per year of coronary heart disease events within two to five years and provide a rationale for intensifying therapy."

Want more data? In a study of calcium scoring CT scans performed on over 8,800 patients, none had known heart disease at the outset. When the subjects were followed up just three years later, the 25% of subjects with the highest calcium CT scores were four times as likely to suffer a heart attack or die from heart disease as those in the lowest 25% of scores. They were also an astounding 26 times more likely to require a stent or bypass operation during that period.

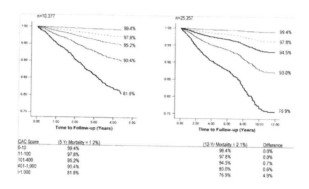

Figure 9. Mortality rates at five and 12 years in patients with low and high calcium scores

At a recent meeting of the American College of Cardiology, several new studies were presented using these scans and important lessons were learned. These included:

1) In a study of nearly 1,000 people tracked for an average of seven years, researchers at Houston Methodist Hospital in Texas found coronary calcium scores were significantly better at predicting cardiac events than two other heart disease tests: the Framingham 10-year risk calculator and the exercise treadmill test. The advantages of calcium scoring were especially prominent in the approximately 80% of participating patients considered to be at low risk for heart disease based on their treadmill test

results. The researchers said that calcium scoring can help catch patients who are on the way to developing heart disease earlier than other available tests.

2) In a 20-year study of nearly 5,600 people, researchers at UCLA Medical Center found that even patients with low calcium scores (1-99) were 50% more likely to die than patients with a calcium score of zero. Moderate scores (100-399) were associated with an 80% greater likelihood of dying and high scores (above 400) were associated with a 300% greater risk of dying as compared to patients with zero calcium. You want to be a zero.

What are your chances of having a normal coronary calcium scan? This will depend on your own established risk factor profile; and it is less likely to be zero if you smoke, are overweight, have pre-diabetes or diabetes or have a high cholesterol or blood pressure. To give you some perspective overall, however, I am involved in a registry of approximately 82,000 persons who recently underwent coronary calcium scans. Only 42% had the lowest risk score of zero. There were 31% of subjects scoring between

1-99, 16% were between 100-399 and were considered to indicate high risk, and finally 11% scored greater than 400 and are at very high risk. There were 2,801 persons that had the extreme score of greater than 1,000. Therefore, it's about 60% likely that you will have some coronary calcification but until the score is determined, the overall predictive significance is nothing more than guesswork.

Can the abnormal coronary calcium score be treated? I will go into much more detail on this in a future chapter. However, a study of 1,005 patients with an abnormal coronary calcium score were treated with aspirin and some with a statin to lower their cholesterol. The average score was 370 units. After four years of treatment, follow-up patients who received a statin had a 7% rate of heart events, such as a heart attack, versus 12% of those which received a placebo. There need to be more studies geared towards determining how the risk can be lowered by specific treatments; however, this study gives a glimpse of the power of finding and treating silent heart disease an early stage.

The American College of Cardiology, of which I am a member and

Fellow, took a big step forward in 2011 when they commented on coronary calcium CT scans. They released new guidelines for assessment of CV risk in asymptomatic adults. Based on evidence from a very large number of studies in more than 100,000 patients, the new guidelines contain two Class IIa indications for calcium CT scans. The American College of Cardiology defines Class IIa indications as those for which "[t]he weight of evidence or opinion is in favor of the procedure or treatment." The Class IIa indications for coronary calcium CT scans are for asymptomatic patients with an intermediate (10% to 20%) 10-year risk of cardiac events, based on the Framingham risk score or other global risk algorithms, as well as for asymptomatic patients 40 years and older with diabetes mellitus. Because the number of US adults with an intermediate FRS and/or diabetes is substantial, these guidelines mean that many persons should have coronary CT calcium scanning.

"Bulletproof Your Heart" Summary

1. Silent dangerous plaque in heart arteries is almost always calcified

2. CT scanners can detect and measure this silent killer in seconds

3. A score of zero predicts a very low score; anything higher is a risk

4. Treatment can lower the risk of a heart attack if heart arteries are calcified

ACTION STEP

If you have never had a coronary artery calcium CT scan and do not know if you are walking around with dangerous plaque, call your local hospitals now. Find out who has the fastest CT machine, remembering that a 256 slice CT is faster than a 64 slice machine, and so on. A FLASH CT scanner may be the fastest imaging choice if you can find one with low radiation levels. You can ask how many mSv are used for this quick exam at various hospitals and pick the lowest result. Find out if the cost is out of pocket, remembering it should be about $200 or less, and find out if you need a physician's prescription. If you do, talk to your doctor and ask for one. In fact, give your health care provider a copy of this book and tell them to get one also. Finally, remember the vitamin pack you can order for radiation safety preparation. As Nike says, JUST DO IT!

Now that you have a clearer understanding of the importance of scans,

be sure to log onto

Visit www.drjoelkahn.com/deadexecs OR

Text **PREVENT** to 58885 OR

You can text your email address to 248-731-5145

On the website, you will find a video series that will walk you through

stress management and breathing techniques you can easily implement

into your busy schedule. You'll also find a PDF file to bring with you to

your scheduled doctor appointment entitled, "Questions to Ask Your

Doctor".

Chapter 5

Carotid Imaging: Thick is Sick and Thin is In

> *"The world is changing very fast. Big will not beat small anymore."*
>
> **Rupert Murdoch, CEO of 21st Century Fox**

Denise prided herself on researching the latest in medical advances and her reading indicated that a healthy mouth was necessary for a healthy body. She learned that just two miles from her home, there was an expert in gum disease and periodontal disease and that this dentist actually lectured to other dentists all over the country. She scheduled an appointment on a day that her commitments to her family food wholesale business were lighter than usual. Since the death of her husband, she had been running the business single-handedly and a few of her prior healthy habits had slipped away. She had to admit that she made too many excuses for her diet and lack of sleep. She was impressed by the dentist's careful description of the connection between gum disease and heart health and she permitted him to test for some advanced markers of periodontal health. On her return visit, she learned that she had a genetic marker indicating that she was producing an inflammatory agent called interleukin 6 (IL-6) at above average rates, putting her mouth and arteries at risk. Her specialist told her that he was concerned that this indicated an increased risk of artery damage and that a simple ultrasound performed on her neck arteries with special software could identify whether her arteries were appropriate for her age, or indicated silent signs of advanced artery aging. Although she would have to pay for this exam, she consented and eagerly awaited the results of the CIMT (Carotid Intima-Media Thickness) examination. She was concerned to learn that the results indicated that her "vascular age" was five years beyond her birth age. It was enough of a jolt to get her focused on returning to walking 10,000 steps a day, packing healthier lunches for her office days and setting a schedule to get to bed by 10pm so that she could wake up at 5.30am refreshed. At the time of writing, she is currently planning a complete evaluation of her heart attack risk.

By now you are an expert in coronary artery calcium scanning and why this simple task can save your life. I hope that this book has motivated you to search on the web for a local facility and have scheduled your examination, if you have never previously had one. Coronary calcium scanning is not the only technique that is scientifically proven to detect silent artery disease. In fact, when the American College of Cardiology gave a high endorsement to the use of coronary calcium CT scans in 2011, they also mentioned another technique, called CIMT scanning. The advantage of the CIMT scan is that it uses ultrasound, not radiation. Therefore, there can be no argument about safety; it's the same technology used for imaging pregnant mothers, for example. Furthermore, I hesitate to repeat the coronary calcium CT scan more than every five to 10 years because of the issue of radiation. A CIMT scan, however, can be done on a repeated basis and can be used to "know your score" and

actually determine if silent plaque is advancing or regressing. There are

hundreds of scientific studies documenting the unique information that

this kind of scan gives about the presence of silent plaque in one of the

major arteries of the body, the carotid artery, which leads directly to the

brain. You should learn more about this technique and in this chapter, I

will outline why it is an integral part of my clinical practice, which may

help you to live a heart attack- and stroke-free life.

The use of the ultrasound CIMT has been around since the 1980s

and requires sophisticated software not normally found in hospitals and

clinics. It provides an analysis of very subtle measurements obtained by

imaging the carotid artery, which although it sounds complicated, actually

constitutes a very simple examination. An ultrasound probe is placed first

on one side of the neck and then the other, and images are made of the

carotid artery. This is painless and generally quite rapid. It's similar to the

ultrasound done in many hospitals looking for established plaque or actual

advanced narrowing of carotid arteries. In fact, if a CIMT scan is planned in an individual without known heart or vascular disease and an established plaque or narrowing is found, there is no need to do the advanced CIMT measurements. The scan will have identified without doubt that the patient is suffering from advanced arterial damage and aggressive measures to stop and reverse vascular damage, as will be explained later in this manual, need to be implemented as soon as possible. However, the CIMT is unique in that it provides an analysis beyond the visual presence of plaque by using very sophisticated measurements which are low-cost, comfortable, without the need of any intravenous access or injection and without any radiation.

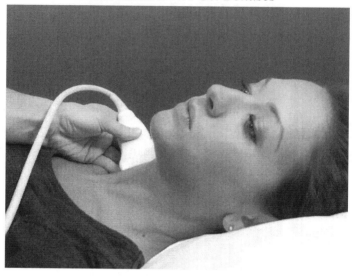

Figure 10. The ultrasound procedure of obtaining a CIMT

What is being measured? The inner lining of any artery, known as the intima, is very thin, while the next layer of an artery further outside the blood flow lumen is called the media. The two together make up a thickness defined as the intima-media thickness. As atherosclerosis develops in an artery, the first evidence of damage is seen in a condensing of the intima-media thickness, caused by various components of damage. The CIMT software measures in millimeters the thickness of these two inner walls of the artery and can determine if soft plaque is accumulating. It can measure precisely how much plaque (invisible to the usual methods of analysis and interpretation) is present. There are large databases involving thousands of patients reporting normal values for the CIMT by age and gender for comparison. There is also a group of studies which determine the average progression of this CIMT measurement from year to year as we age. If the CIMT measurement is progressing faster than the average rate, soft plaque is developing in the carotid and all of the other arteries in the body at a more rapid pace. Therefore, major attempts at preventive strategies need to be instituted. On the other hand, it can be documented that the CIMT actually regresses with measures aimed at lifestyle, supplements and other treatments. This can be one of the earliest and safest ways to assess your arteries over time and your risk for heart and vascular disease. My recommendation is that if you don't want to be a dead exec, you get an initial CIMT and you follow it up over time with subsequent scans, so that you can track your progress while you're working on your lifestyle. Remember, the initial sign of vascular disease in 50% of people is sudden death - so don't delay.

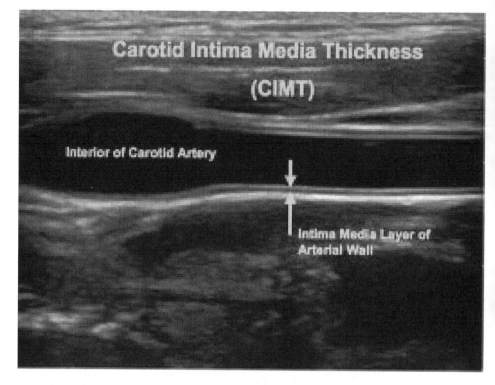

Figure 11. An example of a CIMT ultrasound image

Want some more details about CIMT? In healthy middle-aged

persons, the CIMT at the level of the common carotid artery measures

about 0.6-0.7 millimeters. The thickness increases with age and is

generally thicker in men than in women. Using the normal databases

which are published in the medical literature, one way of reporting the

results is that less than the 25th percentile for age and gender would be ow risk, 25th to 75th percentile is considered the average thickness, while finally those that are more than the 75th percentile for age have the thickest arteries with the most increased cardiovascular risk.

Many studies have established that the CIMT measurement is a marker of silent atherosclerosis. The thickness is associated with the known risk factors for atherosclerosis, such as smoking and diabetes. A number of studies have examined the relationship between the CIMT measurement and future risk of events, such as heart attack, stroke and death. For example, in 2007, a systematic review of eight large population studies reported on the ability of CIMT to predict future cardiovascular events. There were over 37,000 subjects followed for over five years. For every 0.1 micrometer increase in CIMT, the risk of heart attack increased by 10% to 15% and the risk of stroke increased by 13% to 18%.

The Rotterdam study was a single center follow-up of almost 8,000 individuals older than 55 years old. Stroke risk increased gradually with increasing CIMT. Similarly, heart attack risk increased in a comparatively linear way, as well. The CIMT allowed a prediction that some individuals were at 1 ½ times the risk of heart attack than the average.

As mentioned in the previous section, the American College of Cardiology and the American Heart Association guidelines which were recently published found enough evidence for imaging of silent atherosclerosis, including the use of CIMT imaging, to recommend their application for cardiovascular risk assessment. The assessment was given a level IIa recommendation, similar to the coronary artery calcium scanning.

What makes the CIMT increase? A number of studies link increased CIMT thickness to age. However, other markers measured by preventive doctors are also related to the thickness of the CIMT. A marker of inflammation called the C-reactive protein (or CRP) is related to the thickness of the carotid artery. Identifying and controlling inflammation - as will be discussed in the following chapter - is crucial. Fibrinogen is a marker of both inflammation and blood clotting which can easily be measured; there is also a relationship between elevated fibrinogen and increased CIMT measurements.

What has been learned about slowing the rate of CIMT progression? This general topic will be discussed later in this book, but studies have shown that by using serial CIMT measurements, treatments can slow down or even reverse the progression. Cholesterol-lowering medicines such as statins and other medicines including niacin have been shown to delay CIMT progression. In a recent publication following patients for 20 years, treatment was found to reduce Carotid Intima-Media Thickness. The treatment included a combination of statins, niacin and colestipol.

At the present time, CIMT measurements are not covered by insurance in most states and clinics offer this examination for around $200-$250. These scans can be repeated over time to allow accurate measurement of progression or regression of plaque. The best summary of the use of CIMT is probably the statement by the American College of Cardiology in 2011 indicating that "measurement of carotid artery intima-media thickness is reasonable for cardiovascular risk assessment in asymptomatic adults at intermediate risk."

"Bulletproof Your Heart" Summary

1. Thickening of the lining of arteries to the brain is a marker of silent damage

2. A simple ultrasound called a CIMT exam can be done to measure this

3. The thicker the CIMT, the more the disease is developing and the higher the risk

4. The CIMT ultrasound can be repeated to learn if arteries are healing with therapy

<u>ACTION STEP</u>

Try to find a high-quality center offering CIMT in your area. It is worth the effort because over the years, it can provide a window to the health of your arteries and provide feedback on your heart attack and stroke prevention program.

Visit www.drjoelkahn.com/deadexecs OR

Text **PREVENT** to 58885 OR

You can text your email address to 248-731-5145

On the website, you will find a video series that will walk you through stress management and breathing techniques you can easily implement into your busy schedule. You'll also find a PDF file to bring with you to your scheduled doctor appointment entitled, "Questions to Ask Your Doctor".

Chapter 6

Get Life-Saving Lab Tests

"When you innovate, you've got to be prepared for everyone

telling you you're nuts."

Larry Ellison, CEO of Oracle

I do not have just one case study to share here; I have hundreds of patients who have come to me with the same statement: "My doctor told me that my heart attack [or my stroke, my stent, my bypass surgery, my leg bypass] is completely unexplained and that I am a freak of medicine; no one can figure me out." Their names are Ted, Tina, Sam and Samantha, and there are a lot of them. However, I am sorry; you simply do NOT have these life threatening events at the age of 43, or 37, or 62 or even 74, without an explanation. It may be a lifestyle issue not yet probed, like secretive smoking habits or use of illicit drugs like cocaine, but more commonly it is a previously untested biochemical or genetic abnormality. We have a long way to go to completely understand heart disease, but over 300 factors have been linked to heart attacks and strokes and many can be tested at an advanced heart attack prevention clinic. Is it your homocysteine level? Your MTHFR status? Your lipoprotein(a)? Your clotting factors? Your insulin resistance? The list goes on and on and on. Make no mistake, the common lifestyle habits such as smoking, eating processed foods, gaining weight, skipping exercise and excessive stress with poor management skills and subsequent poor sleep, are the main factors to blame. But if you are one of those vulnerable to some of the less obvious heart attack risk factors which can be measured and modified, wouldn't you want to know? I hope you read on with interest about your health.

If you want to prevent a heart attack and enjoy your executive position (and your life beyond the C-suite) in great heart health, you do not want routine lab tests, you want C-suite lab tests! They can tell so much more about the state of your heart and the risk of a heart attack. Just like the car wash at the gas station offers the standard and the supreme car wash, with the supreme offering all the extra treatments for preserving the beauty of your car, "supreme" labs can reveal metabolic and genetic abnormalities that can be addressed and may influence your chances of developing heart issues. You are certainly worth the same care your car gets. The list below are services often offered by some specialty laboratory providers like Cleveland Heart Labs, Boston Heart Labs, Spectracell and others. These are part of the tools which I use to make my patients reach heart attack-proof status. An outline of the services are provided below, but don't worry too much about the minor details; just make sure you get checked thoroughly.

Advanced cholesterol panels. You've probably been told to keep your total cholesterol below 200 and your LDL-cholesterol below 100 mg/dl. In addition to knowing that basic information, you also want to know the advanced LDL particle number and size. Two patients could both have identical cholesterol scores and still be at vastly different levels of risk of heart disease. One of those patients might be overweight, consume a diet rich in processed foods full of fat and sugar, be sedentary and sleep poorly. The other might be trim, use the gym four times a week, consume five to 10 servings of organic fruits and vegetables most days and sleep deeply for seven hours a night. The first patient might have an LDL particle number of 2,150, while the second patient's number is 980. Ideal LDL particle numbers are around 1,000 or less, and increases above that are predictive of atherosclerosis and events like heart attacks and strokes. So obviously, 980 trumps 2,150 - but there is no way of knowing that information without the right blood test. So the routine total cholesterol and LDL numbers alone are simply not good enough. All LDL cholesterol is dangerous when elevated; the advanced cholesterol labs just help define exactly how dangerous it is by reporting the LDL particle number and size of the LDL particles. Large LDL particle sizes may be somewhat less injurious than small, dense LDL particles. You need to know the details for CARE-full advice. Finally, LDL cholesterol may be most injurious to your arteries when they become affected by rusting, or oxidation. Oxidized

LDL cholesterol levels can be measured and attempts to lower oxidation

by lifestyle management (eat your damn vegetables and berries!) should

be instituted.

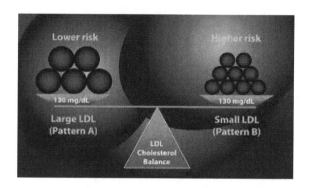

Figure 12. Advanced cholesterol tests measure LDL particle

number

High sensitivity C-reactive protein. Inflammation is a fire that

slowly erodes blood vessels; C-reactive protein is a marker for

inflammation. In the past decade, a test for high sensitivity C-reactive

protein (hs-CRP) has changed the assessment of patients dramatically. If

your hs-CRP is normal (usually under 1.0 mg/dl), your arteries do not

appear to be have become inflamed by your diet, lifestyle, waistline or other factors. On the other hand, if your hs-CRP is elevated (anything from 1 mg/dl all the way to over 20), something is wrong with your lifestyle or health and major efforts to identify and correct problems need to be pursued. I order this exam on every patient at least once a year. If the results are abnormal, I search for a bad diet and lack of exercise along with unexpected sites of inflammation. I ask about dental, prostate, urinary and bowel infections that may represent the subtle root cause.

Homocysteine and MTHFR status. About 40 years ago, an astute doctor observed early artery damage in young children who had an elevated level of a naturally-occurring amino acid called homocysteine. Research led to identifying a very complex series of chemical reactions in the body which deal with amino acid metabolism, a process called methylation. Certain vitamins make these cycles function properly. In adults, increased levels of homocysteine have also been associated with increased risk of vascular damage. At a minimum, measuring homocysteine levels reflects the status of the methylation process in the body, so it's a very important way to regulate gene function. Patients with high levels of homocysteine can be treated with B complex vitamins, which is a pretty simple solution. A safe homocysteine level is under 10 umol/L, and an even better level is under 8 umol/L. I get very concerned when it is in the high teens or over 20 umol/L. If the homocysteine levels are abnormal, the genetic root cause can assessed by determining whether your parents gave you normal or abnormal genes, called MTHFR genes. You may have two normal genes, one normal and one abnormal, or two abnormal genes (10% of the population have two abnormal MTHFR 677 genes). If your genes are abnormal, you can return the metabolism of folate to normal by eating lots of folate-rich foods (greens) and taking special B complex vitamins that are "methylated" to overcome the genetic trap you were born with.

Lipoprotein(a). Lipoprotein(a), or Lpa, is an inherited form of the LDL cholesterol bound to a special protein. Much research has connected high levels of Lpa to early cardiovascular disease. This is a widely available blood test. I draw it on my patients if they have an abnormal calcium score or a thick carotid artery, as well as anyone with any sign of heart disease at a young age. High levels can be treated with niacin, hormone replacement and vitamins. Most labs indicate a normal Lpa is under 30 mg/dl, but I have seen readings all the way to 200 mg/dl. If you test high, consider it as an opportunity to incorporate lifestyle changes which will lower the LDL cholesterol particle number to acceptable levels, while also lowering the Lpa level.

Fasting blood sugar, insulin, hemoglobin A1C and a two-hour glucose tolerance test. Diabetes is a horrible diagnosis. So often doctors are disinterested about the new diagnosis because it is literally a dime a dozen to see it; however, it may rob a dozen years from your life and greatly increase your chances of a heart attack. Any standard blood panel will check your fasting blood sugar. Doctors may not worry you until your blood sugar is in the diabetic range of more than 120 mg/dl, but studies suggest that a fasting blood sugar of less than 85 mg/dl is optimal. Each jump above 85 increases the risk of aging and vessel injury significantly. Blood sugar, however, only shows you half of the equation because the blood sugar is regulated by insulin. If the level of insulin is elevated, the pancreas is working "overtime" to maintain blood sugar and the arteries are at risk. If both the fasting blood sugar and the fasting insulin are normal, glucose metabolism is normal. I also often order a hemoglobin A1C to look at average blood sugar levels over the last two to three months and a two-hour glucose tolerance test using a drink of sugar-rich liquid to completely assess for pre-diabetes.

Vitamin D. The interest in the connection between Vitamin D and healthy arteries is rapidly expanding. A low Vitamin D level has been connected to high blood pressure, arterial damage, congestive heart failure, poor brain health and other important problems. Normally Vitamin D is obtained by sunlight and foods such as mushrooms; however, even in sunny areas, most people test low. African-Americans are especially at risk for Vitamin D deficiency due to darker skin color, which blocks sunlight from making the vitamin in the skin. Ask your doctor to check your level. You want your blood level of D to be over 30 ng/ml and optimally 50-80 ng/ml.

Uric acid levels and GGT. These two simple and older blood examinations are coming back in use as they provide unique insight into the health of the cardiovascular system. Uric acid is produced from energy products like ATP and an elevated level is linked to cardiovascular damage. GGT is a liver enzyme which may indicate an overall poor functioning of cell membranes in the liver and provide an insight to the overall health of your metabolism. Normal uric acid levels are 4-8 mg/dl and levels over 10 are concerning. Normal levels of GGT are under 50 IU/L and levels over 100 IU/L are concerning for generalized cell membrane dysfunction.

Thyroid hormones. Many environmental toxins affect the thyroid gland, especially endocrine disruptors such as plastics and personal care items like toothpaste. An advanced thyroid panel will include the TSH, free T4, free T3 and the TPO antibodies. The ideal TSH to avoid subclinical hypothyroidism (underactive thyroid) is to have a TSH under 2.5 mIU/L. The normal range for the other tests will vary by the lab.

Sex hormones. If you are a man, make sure the lab measures total and free testosterone, DHEAs and estradiol levels. If you are a woman, learn the same labs results along with progesterone levels.

Additional genetic tests. We are at the beginning of a new era of determining your genetic make-up by simple blood tests or swabs of cells from your inner mouth and characterizing how you are wired for metabolism. For example, you can find out right now if you are metabolizing caffeine slowly or quickly, have a genetic issue with gluten, Vitamin C and saturated fats and you can be examined for the 9p21 gene, which may predict double the risk of heart attack. Another genetic assay, for the cholesterol-carrying particle apolipoprotein E, predicts a risk of Alzheimer's disease and indicates if a low-fat, vegetable-based diet low in alcohol is the preferred menu for your genetic makeup.

Telomere length assessment. Do you know what a telomere is? Probably, you have been busy running your company and not focusing so much on recent Nobel Prize awards for Medicine. One of the most exciting areas of aging research is on the importance of the length of the tips of your chromosomes, called telomeres. The Nobel Prize in Medicine was awarded to three scientists in 2009 for describing an enzyme, named telomerase, which can add length to telomeres and holds the potential to slow or reverse aging. Does this matter? It does; because every year, as cells replicate, the tips of your chromosomes get shorter and shorter. In fact, it is estimated that at conception your telomere caps have 15,000 "base pairs" and that by birth you are down to 10,000 base pairs due to rapid replication during pregnancy. Then you lose maybe 100-150 base pairs each year as you grow and age. One theory of aging is that when telomeres get short enough, the cell dies. When enough cells die, so do you. Gruesome - but how do you find out where you stand?

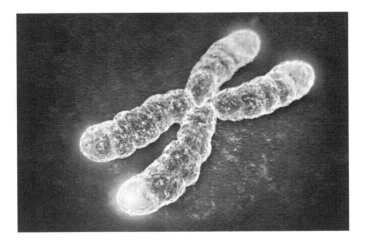

Figure 13. A chromosome showing the tips, or telomeres, in green

Several reputable companies have tests to measure your average and shortest telomere length. I had mine checked and so can you too. If you want to know your true genetic age, you can find out. It may show you are younger inside than the number of candles on your cake... or it may say the opposite. Either way, you can use the information to plan your lifestyle/career balance.

"Bulletproof Your Heart" Summary

1. Advanced cholesterol profiles give much more information about your risk

2. Arteries can be damaged by other abnormalities, which can be measured

3. Genetic markers like MTHFR and APOE can be measured

4. Your true genetic age is assessed by measuring your telomere length

ACTION STEPS

Lab tests are a vital part of your care. Be sure to find a health care provider which offers advanced lab testing and can explain the tests in an understandable manner. More information can pinpoint your risk.

If heading to the lab creates stress in your life, be sure to take advantage

of the bonus techniques by logging onto

Visit www.drjoelkahn.com/deadexecs OR

Text **PREVENT** to 58885 OR

You can text your email address to 248-731-5145

On the website, you will find a video series that will walk you through

stress management and breathing techniques you can easily implement

into your busy schedule. You'll also find a PDF file to bring with you to

your scheduled doctor appointment entitled, "Questions to Ask Your

Doctor".

Chapter 7

True Causes of Disease

> *"To build a great a great company, which is a CEO's job, sometimes you have to stand up against the conventional wisdom."*
>
> **Carly Fiorina, CEO Hewlett-Packard**

My heart went out to Sandy when she trudged slowly into my office for a consultation. She had come for assistance with her blood pressure, which had been difficult to control for the past year. She had read that I used an integrative approach. Although she had no known heart disease, I was impressed by her medicine list of 12 prescription drugs and the equally long list of her specialists: rheumatology for joint pains, neurology for tingling leg pains, endocrinology for her blood sugar, gastroenterology for her reflux, and so on. A more thorough history revealed that she had assumed VP of Sales for her family marketing business, which had grown to involve multiple offices in multiple states. She was on an airplane at least twice a week. In her late 50s, she was worn out and was looking for a quick fix. She admitted that she felt 20 years older than her driver's license age. A review of her lifestyle indicated that at least half of the meals she ate every week were on the run, often in airports or hotel lobbies. She averaged five hours of sleep a night. Her exercise program had dwindled to treadmill time at home on weekends only. She grabbed for diet sodas more than ever and often ate protein health bars for a breakfast on the run. During this past year, she had gained 14 pounds and the three blood pressure medicines she was taking were failing to control her pressure. She was looking at her watch and asked me if I knew of a better pill or supplement she could add to her current mix to lower her blood pressure. I looked at my watch, realized I did have a rare extra 30 minutes overlapping with my lunch break, and we talked. I told her that words like diabetes, arthritis, obesity and hypertension were diagnoses that fit neatly into billing codes and research papers - but they were not causes. We talked about the fact that most or all of her ills and pills were due to her lifestyle. The poor sleep; the suboptimal diet; the high stress without adaptive strategies; the inadequate movement; the chemicals she was drinking and applying to her body and clothes; the likelihood that she had food intolerances... these were the causes of her woes. Although I had to add some supplements (magnesium, a probiotic and flax seed powder) to help her with her blood pressure, I referred her to a holistic nutritionist and a trainer who also did life coaching. I told her if she would work at the root causes of her unacceptable health (which was on a collision course with a heart attack, stroke or cancer), she would be able to stop using most or all of her medicines.

Here is an easy question any executive can nail: what is the leading cause of death in the Western world? As a former chairman of the American Heart Association and executive leadership member there, I hope we have done our job in educating the public to point out to you that the answer is HEART DISEASE. Much earlier in the introduction of this book, I reviewed the scary and disturbing statistics . The University of

Michigan Big House, my alma mater, is 45 minutes west of my office and

holds over 100,000 fans. Imagine filling that stadium seven times - over

700,000 men and women, some in their 20s or even younger - to get a

grasp on the number of heart attacks yearly in the US alone. So yes, in a

sense, heart disease is the leading cause of death in the Western world.

Except, that is not actually correct. In a landmark paper entitled

Actual causes of Death in the United States published in 1993 by

McGinnis and Foege, these researchers from the CDC in Atlanta dared to

stand up against conventional wisdom. They analyzed the 2,148,000

deaths in the US in 1990, 720,000 of which were attributed to heart

disease. They measured lifestyle habits which had contributed to these

deaths; the root causes. They found that smoking, followed by poor diet

and inadequate activity, were the three most common actual causes of

disease and death - all factors which are modifiable. Their data indicated

that a new robotic procedure or a designer pill will never have the hope of

improving health as much as focusing on lifestyle choices. They recognized that "the three leading causes of death-tobacco, diet and activity patterns, are all rooted in behavioral choices. Behavioral change is motivated not by knowledge alone, but also by a supportive social environment and the availability of facilitative services." My colleague and friend Dr. David Katz, Professor of Medicine and founding director of Yale's Prevention Medicine Center, lectures that your use of your feet, fork and fingers (smoking) will determine your fate. Individuals motivated and determined to have a career free of heart disease need to appreciate the power of these three F's.

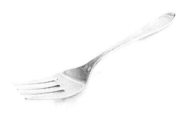

Figure 14. The fork is the most powerful tool in preventing heart attacks

Maybe you are saying that was 1993 and so much has changed in our lives, given that was even before iPads and crowdsourcing. In 2004, researchers at the CDC analyzed the data from deaths in the US in 2000 to provide an updated analyses of actual causes of death. Once again, in over two million deaths, heart disease was the leading diagnosis. But Mokdad and his colleagues found that smoking, followed by poor diet and inadequate activity, were the largest actual causes of deaths, accounting for over half of all deaths. The next most important lifestyle factor, alcohol abuse, was a distant fourth. The only difference in the decade since McGinnis and Foege shared their novel analysis was that the tobacco use had fallen slightly and the combination of poor diet and inadequate physical activity had climbed as a true cause of death by 2000.

By now, you may still have not yet completely bought into the idea that the path you need to follow to live a heart attack-free life will require daily attention to your feet, fork and fingers. Fast forward medical research to 2009, when Dr. Earl Ford from the Centers for Disease Control and Prevention (CDC), along with colleagues in Germany, analyzed almost 30,000 residents of Potsdam over an eight-year period for the development of potentially career-ending diagnoses like heart attacks, diabetes, strokes and cancer. They found four factors which strongly predicted avoiding these monumental illnesses. Was it their genetics, predestined to have illness? In fact, the four factors which protected residents from disease were: never smoking, maintaining an optimal weight, regular physical activity (averaging 30 minutes a day) and finally eating a diet rich in fruits, vegetables and whole grains which was low in meat. Of the total population, 9% practiced all four health factors. Those 9% had a dramatically lower risk of developing a chronic disease. How dramatic? The risk of developing diabetes was 93% lower, heart attacks 81% lower, stroke 50% lower and cancer 36% lower. They concluded that "adhering to four simple healthy lifestyle factors can have a strong impact on the prevention of chronic diseases." Admittedly, it is possible to choose not to smoke, to exercise, to eat mainly fruits, vegetables and whole grains with little meat on a daily basis. These are simply the three F's again... but optimal weight? Weight is not a behavioral habit, but is rather a combination of calories in, calories out, genetic inputs, cultural forces, the health of your intestinal "microbiome", stress and other factors. However, the emphasis to maintain a trim weight and waist is an important lesson.

It may be a bit over the top to throw one more piece of research at you, but I do not think you can hear "Feet, forks, fingers!" too often in a world which screams "Sit, sundaes, smoke!" Earl Ford, MD, still at the CDC, looked at deaths in Alameda County, California, and published data on real causes of death in 2012. Over 8,000 residents were followed and 745 deaths occurred during six years of follow-up. Although heart disease was the number one most common official cause of death, Dr. Ford found that once again smoking, physical inactivity and poor diet were the most common actual causes of fatal disease conditions. Residents who didn't smoke, who exercised an average of 30 minutes a day and who ate diets rich in fruits, vegetables and grains had a risk of dying that was 82% less than those who ignored these habits.

The message is clear; from 1993 to 2012, the data is clear. Dead execs are most likely to get that way by smoking, eating a diet that is not high in fruits, vegetables and whole grains and skipping exercise. Add in excess weight as a fourth factor and a perfect storm is created for suffering from fatal heart attacks, strokes, diabetes and cancer. You simply can't afford to ignore this overwhelming information. It is not a laser, a space-age operating suite or a robotic surgery module which has the best chance of protecting your health. Lifestyle medicine is the most powerful and proven way to avoid falling over the waterfall into the abyss below and requiring the acute care medical system which may successfully rescue you and patch you back together with the marvels of modern medicine... or may fail to do this. Every meal matters; every cigarette matters; every minute of activity matters. Don't wait until retirement to make these simple habits part of your daily rituals - you may not even make it to retirement if you ignore these powerful practices! In fact, make them part of the culture of your corporation and have all employees commit to not smoking, provide healthy foods rich in produce and grains in cafeterias and vending machines and build standing desks, walking meetings and gym memberships into the daily rituals. To life!

"Bulletproof Your Heart" Summary

Heart disease is the number one diagnosis for deaths in the Western world - but it is not the number one cause of death. The true causes of cardiac deaths are:

1. Smoking

2. Diets low in fruits, vegetables and whole grains

3. Inadequate physical activity

4. Excess body weight and waist measurements

ACTION STEP

Seek out every method of quitting smoking, whether it be prescription drugs, patches, chewing gum, electronic cigarettes, hypnosis, acupuncture or group therapy, and do them all again and again until you quit. Add in fruits and vegetables along with whole grains at every meal. Buy a pedometer and start measuring how many steps a day you take. Slowly build up to 10,000 as a goal, if you are able. You can save your life with the three F's.

And, if all else fails in your attempts to quit smoking, be sure to take

advantage of the bonus techniques which will help reduce day-to-day

stress and which can be implemented just about anywhere, by logging

onto

Visit www.drjoelkahn.com/deadexecs OR

Text **PREVENT** to 58885 OR

You can text your email address to 248-731-5145

On the website, you will find a video series that will walk you through

stress management and breathing techniques you can easily implement

into your busy schedule. You'll also find a PDFile to bring with you to

your scheduled doctor appointment entitled, "Questions to Ask Your

Doctor".

Chapter 8

Manage Stress or Lose

"Remaining disciplined by managing both time and productivity well is

the backbone to good stress management."

John Benson, CEO of eFinancialCareers.com

Debbie was scared when I met her in the emergency room; she was sweating and suffering intense chest pressure. A 52-year-old communications company executive, she had been rushed to the hospital from her home after calling the emergency services when the symptoms started, 45 minutes earlier. She had no heart history. She indicated between sobs that she had just left the funeral of a childhood friend a few hours before her symptoms began. I looked at her ECG and it was clear she was suffering an acute heart attack. Within minutes, we were in the cardiac

catheterization laboratory and beginning an angiogram procedure. By

carefully injecting contrast material into her three heart arteries, I soon

detected that she did not have the usual blockages seen in almost every

other heart attack suffering. When I took a picture of her heart strength,

she had a large area of weakened heart muscle, the hallmark of a heart

attack... but no blockage. She was a classic example of a stress-induced

syndrome called the Broken Heart Syndrome. Fortunately, Debbie was

discharged home within two days and studies of her heart strength two

weeks later demonstrated a total return of her heart pump function to

normal levels. I asked her to study methods of managing stress and I was

gratified to learn on subsequent office visits that she was regularly

practicing meditation.

Without question, emotions can have an impact on the heart. Why

do we smoke? Why do we skip our workouts? Why do we reach for

donuts and french fries when we know they are a fast track to disease and

death? Often the answer is poor stress management. Stress can kill. The underlying cause of the "true causes" discussed in Chapter 7 is often

inadequate attention to stress. It is estimated that 75% of doctor visits have

their root cause in stress or the ways we deal with stress, in terms of poor

habits. For executives, the number may even be higher due to overloaded

work schedules, excessive travel and deadlines.

Stress cannot be avoided, but it can be managed with proven

techniques. For example, relaxation strategies and respiratory training can

add vitality and wellbeing. Sadly, in traditional medicine, the focus is

often only on the body and little attention is paid to the mind or the spirit.

Fortunately, the tide is turning as yoga, meditation and tai chi are showing

up in health clubs and even many corporate wellness programs.

Why am I so certain that stress and emotions can harm your heart

or even put you at risk of death? Stress was described as a medical

condition in the 1950s by a Hungarian-born physician named Hans Selye,

MD, working in Montreal. He wrote several ground-breaking books,

including Stress Without Distress, and founded the Canadian Institute of

Stress. In the 1970s, Dr. Meyer Friedman, a cardiologist, introduced the terminology of Type A behavior in chronically impatient and stressed persons. His research indicated that Type A patients had an increased risk of heart disease and heart attacks. Although these important pioneers opened doors and minds about the role of stress in heart disease, it was the observation of a new syndrome in the last 20 years which began to convince the medical community that stress, a difficult entity to measure, was a powerful cause of heart disease. This new syndrome has been called the Broken Heart Syndrome, or stress cardiomyopathy, and is what Debbie suffered in the case study. First described in Japan, the classic case involves someone who learns of terrible news which results in strong emotions. A death of a loved one, a car accident or a child who reveals an alcoholic problem are some examples I have seen. During this strong response (which might manifest itself in sobbing or screaming), chest pressure develops in the patient, often accompanied by shortness of breath and profuse perspiration, just like a typical heart attack. These women (yes, it can be a man but it's much less common) are rushed to the emergency department and their electrocardiogram looks like a classic large heart attack. They are then rushed to the catheterization laboratory for an emergency angiogram but usually no blockage is found - quite different than the typical heart attack due to a 100% blocked heart artery. There is damage to the heart found on pictures and lab tests. No stent or bypass is needed and with medication the damage usually completely resolves itself. However, women with the Broken Heart Syndrome are at risk of suffering from it again if emotions flare. I have had patients with this syndrome who got very upset on the phone over bills, in the bank arguing over mortgage payments and during intense family disputes.

It does not take too much of an imagination to conclude that if stress can be this bad for the heart, strategies which reduce or manage stress must be good for the heart. In fact, the Broken Heart Syndrome is felt to be due to a large surge in adrenaline, the hormone made by the adrenal glands above the kidneys and controlled by the sympathetic nervous system (SNS). Having strategies which reduce the impact of the SNS, and increase the impact of the balancing system called the parasympathetic nervous system PNS, will help you manage your stress, enjoy vitality and hopefully prolong your career and life.

Take yoga, for example; it can be used for stress management and a healthier heart. Yoga is often defined as a union of the mind and body, of motion and breath, of each of us to the other. This is a practice which originated in India but has grown rapidly across the Western world and most communities have access to classes at dedicated studios, fitness centers or even houses of worship. Many online and DVD-based training materials are also available. I even have several yoga training applications on my Smartphone.

There are several styles of yoga. In North America, a style called hatha yoga is most common, including asanas (or flows of movement), pranayamas (or prolonged force of breath) and kriyas (or purification techniques). Generally, there are slower or more intense yoga practices to choose from; some are in warm rooms and some in hot rooms, some geared for athletic individuals and some done even in a chair to allow cardiac patients, older or even infirm persons to participate in at least the breathing practices. The practice of yoga on a regular basis can lead to measurable improvements in flexibility, stamina, muscle strength and

weight control. Measures of the SNS and the PNS show that a regular

practice increases the output of the PNS and decreases the SNS flow,

leading to improvements in a measure of heart function called heart rate

variability. Improvements in heart rate variability occurring with yoga are

suspected to improve actual longevity. Yoga has been shown to increase

insulin release from the pancreas to improve blood sugar control, and has

been shown to lower cholesterol and triglyceride levels when practiced

regularly. While yoga can lower blood pressure, there were not enough

studies to permit a recent American Heart Association panel in 2013 to

scientifically endorse yoga for blood pressure control. The panel did

indicate that there were few risks attached to the practice of yoga, other

than the risk of a musculoskeletal injury. Recent elegant research on gene

expression has shown that a regular yoga practice modifies gene output in

white blood cells and may boost immune health. This would be another

example of epigenetic modification by a healthy lifestyle choice. There

has even been research indicating that when the blood of persons practicing yoga for stress reduction is assayed, there is a higher level of antioxidants. The combination of cardiovascular training, stretching, balance exercises, relaxation and weight-bearing poses to strengthen bones, along with breathing to train improve heart rate variability, make yoga one of the activities which can be done on a daily basis as the sole choice of movement and mind-body activity. I practice yoga regularly.

Meditation is often a part of a yoga practice, but it is also a stand-alone technique that has been extensively studied in patients with cardiovascular disease. Meditation is considered a practice or exercise to increase awareness of consciousness. There are several methods of teaching with transcendental meditation (TM), the most well-known of which were made famous by the Beatles. Mindfulness-based stress reduction (MBSR) as taught by Jon Kabat Zinn, PhD and others is another very popular style. Another style, called the Kirtan Kriya, takes only 12 minutes daily and is a practice which I incorporate into my schedule, often while sitting in a sauna: something I call sauna-tation!

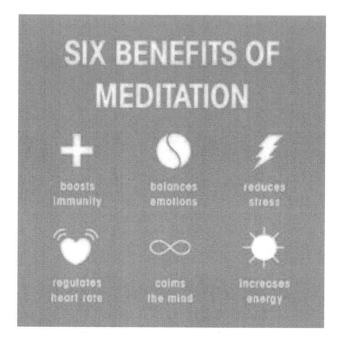

Figure 15. Meditation can improve heart and brain health

Are there documented health benefits to meditative practices?

Meditation does affect the nervous system, even beyond the typical 20-

minute practice one or two times a day, via a mechanism often known as

neuroplasticity. The levels of melatonin have been reported to increase,

perhaps explaining the better sleep which regular meditators describe.

Actual brain volume may even increase, according to research reports.

When measured by EEG recordings, meditation increases brain activity, particularly of the alpha type. Measurements of quality of life and overall health are scored higher in regular meditators than others. During meditation, heart rate and respiratory rate is recorded to drop and the amount of oxygen used by the body decreases. Drops in the stress hormone cortisol, improvements in brain metabolism, stronger immune systems and even measures of slower aging or actual aging reversal have all been documented at University medical centers when meditation has been studied.

One technique which is very easy to use before meetings or in the C-suite is called 4-7-8 breathing and can be done in under 90 seconds. I learned the 4-7-8 breathing practice from the writings of Drs. Andrew Weil and Tieraona Low Dog of the University of Arizona. The technique shifts the autonomic nervous system away from sympathetic predominance (which makes our hearts race and our palms sweaty when we face a stressful situation) and allows the parasympathetic nervous system to shine. 4-7-8 breathing is done by following these simple steps:

1. Sit up straight in a chair.

2. Place the tip of your tongue up against the roof of your mouth. Keep it there through the entire breathing process.

3. Breathe in silently through your nose to the slow count of 4.

4. Hold your breath to the count of 7.

5. Exhale through your mouth to the count of 8, making a slight audible sound.

6. Repeat the 4-7-8 cycle another three times, for a total of four breathing exercises.

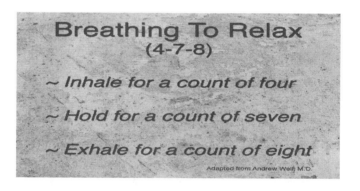

Figure 16. The 4-7-8 breathing technique

Scientific studies indicate that this type of breathing exercise can really work. For example, subjects taught to breathe slowly and deeply as a mind-body practice show beneficial changes in the autonomic nervous system favoring parasympathetic relaxation. They also exhibit increases in skin temperature from better artery flow and reveal reductions in blood pressure, compared to control subjects.

Two additional considerations for stress management during your busy business day include using:

Adaptogens. When I talk to patients about stress, I begin by describing adaptogens, or herbs which appear to be useful in stabilizing physiology and improving anxiety and stress control. I do this because so many of them are already using pills -- typically benzodiazepines like Xanax and Ativan -- and my goal is to get them off those prescription medications as soon as possible.

Frankly, substituting one pill for another is something most patients accept faster than any other technique. I've had success in many patients using L-theanine 200 mg twice a day and ashwagandha 500 mg twice daily, usually together. Even elderly patients report they feel less stressed and more functional. Rhodiola is another adaptogen I like because it has been studied in heart patients and shows benefits for their symptoms. I recommend 100 mg a day.

HeartMath. This is an online program using heart-centered breathing and positive emotions to restore balance between the sympathetic and parasympathetic nervous systems. It requires purchasing a cable that clips on the earlobe and connects to a Smartphone, tablet or PC. I recommend it because it resembles a game, is easy to learn and is supported by published scientific studies showing lower blood pressure, lower cortisol levels, improved memory and better school performance.

"Bulletproof Your Heart" Summary

1. Stress is a response to life situations which raises hormone levels and blood pressure

2. The Broken Heart Syndrome is a dramatic example of stress damaging the heart

3. Management of stress is the key to maintaining healthy heart habits

4. Yoga, meditation, 4-7-8 breathing and HeartMath are proven methods to use

ACTION STEP

Face it, you have daily stress in your life and you may not have a plan to manage it optimally. A good night's sleep, a healthy diet and regular exercise are excellent methods of lessening the impact of stress in the C-suite, so do not skip those healing habits. In addition, learn at least one breathing technique using meditation, HeartMath, yoga or the 4-7-8 sequence to assist you in controlling stress.

Make sure you take advantage of the bonus techniques that will help

reduce day-to-day stress and which can be implemented just about

anywhere, by logging onto

Visit www.drjoelkahn.com/deadexecs OR

Text **PREVENT** to 58885 OR

You can text your email address to 248-731-5145

On the website, you will find a video series that will walk you through

stress management and breathing techniques you can easily implement

into your busy schedule. You'll also find a PDF file to bring with you to

your scheduled doctor appointment entitled, "Questions to Ask Your

Doctor".

Chapter 9

Heart Attacks are CARE-less. Prevent not Stent™

"A man must be big enough to admit his mistakes, smart enough to profit from them and strong enough to correct them."

John C. Maxwell, CEO of The John Maxwell Company

When I saw him (let's call him J), I was impressed. He seemed to actually get it. He shared that in the last five years, he was placing emphasis on sleeping seven hours a night. He ate over seven servings of fruits and vegetables a day, making green smoothies from vegetables many mornings, juicing and adding lentils and beans to most lunches and dinners. In fact, he couldn't remember the last time he had eaten any animal product. He was working out six days a week, mixing up longer group fitness classes before work with some shorter high-intensity fitness

routines, some yoga and some weight training. He never smoked but

admitted he averaged a glass of Pinot noir or Chianti five days a week. His

waist measured 35 inches and had not changed in over 20 years. He had

become a student of meditation and practiced this regularly. Although I

assured him that his risk profile was low (even though he was in his mid

50s), he still wanted more testing. He ran several businesses and was

concerned about the effects of stress and the fact that his father had been

diagnosed with coronary heart disease when he was the same age. He

asked for a coronary artery calcium scan and agreed to prepare for it with

a vitamin packet developed for radiation protection from imaging studies.

Fortunately, the heart scan came back with a zero score and he was

relieved that his risk over the next decade at least was extremely low for a

cardiac event. One last note; this is my autobiography.

There is a mantra that I would like you to repeat over and over.

Heart attacks are preventable. Heart attacks are preventable. Heart attacks

are preventable.

It is that simple. The statistic of one heart attack every 35 seconds; the loss of hundreds of thousands of lives; the cost of billions of dollars... all of this could be reduced by 90%, starting right now, with simple lifestyle measures. And with the advanced measures outlined for you in other chapters, you can push that 90% figure closer to 100%. You NEVER need to suffer a heart attack. A heart attack is CARE-less medical management; make sure you practice CARE-ful management. Spread the word and be the first in your company to master this critical concept.

How can I say that heart attacks are preventable? There is an overwhelming body of science which indicates that this is so. That you haven't heard this before is unfortunate, but it is time to change; the message must be spread. Let's take a brief tour of some medical literature which you should know about and take to heart, literally.

2001

The Harvard School of Public Health reported on a study of 84,941 female nurses followed between 1980-1996. These women were free of heart disease, cancer and diabetes. They provided information on their lifestyle habits and diet. The researchers defined a low-risk lifestyle for disease as a body mass index (weight divided by height) of under 25, a diet high in fiber and polyunsaturated fat while low in trans-fat and glycemic load, regular moderate to vigorous exercise (at least 30 minutes a day), no smoking and drinking at least half an alcoholic drink daily. During follow-up, 3,300 women were diagnosed with diabetes. The single most important predictor of this was being overweight or obese. Sadly, only 3.4% of the almost 85,000 women fit the entire profile of the low risk lifestyle. These women, however, had a 91% lower chance of developing diabetes compared with the other members of the study.

Bottom Line: Diabetes, a major reason people develop heart disease and heart attacks, can be prevented over 90% of the time by managing your lifestyle as well as you manage your business.

2004

The INTERHEART study group evaluated the factors predicting heart attacks in 52 countries. They reported on 15,000 cases of heart attacks and chose the same number of controls. They accumulated data on a host of factors and analyzed which were able to predict developing a heart attack. The found nine risk factors which accounted for 90%-95% of the cases of heart attacks... and all of these factors can be controlled! What were the big nine? The ones you want to identify and eliminate from your life? They were comprised of smoking, elevated ApoB (think bad cholesterol) to ApoA1 (think good cholesterol) ratio, high blood pressure, diabetes, abdominal obesity (waist over 35 inches for a woman and 40 inches for a man), stress, low intake of fruits and vegetables, lower alcohol intake and lack of physical exercise.

Bottom line: The question is, can you take charge of your life and create a lifestyle where you don't smoke, have an occasional glass of red wine, learn stress management techniques like meditation, know and control your blood pressure, cholesterol and blood sugar and trim that waist down? Would that checklist be worth 95% freedom from a heart attack during your career and after?

2006

Harvard researchers analyzed data from 43,000 men in the Health

Professionals Study between the ages of 40-75 who had no heart disease at the outset in 1986. Low-risk men were considered to have a BMI under 25 (normal weight), be non-smokers, be physically active for more than 30 minutes a day, have moderate alcohol intake and have a diet comprised of more than 40% healthy plants. Over the 16 years of follow-up, a heart attack developed in 2,183 men, some of which were fatal heart attacks. Men who had five out of five low risk characteristics had an 87% lower rate of heart attacks! During the study, men who made two or more lifestyle changes to move closer to the ideal low risk group had a lower risk of heart attacks, too.

Bottom line: It is never too late to change, and change should start today. These are five simple steps.

2007

Swedish investigators studied over 24,000 women after menopause who were free of heart disease. 308 cases of heart attacks developed over six years of follow-up. A low risk diet (high scores for fruits and vegetable intake, whole grains, legumes, fish, moderate alcohol intake), along with not smoking, walking or biking 40 minutes daily and maintaining a trim waist-to-hip ratio reduced the risk of heart attacks by... 92%!

Bottom Line: After menopause, women are at increased risk of heart attacks and stroke, but they can be almost completely eliminated by LIFESTYLE MEDICINE. Get on the program and live heart attack-free.

2008

Harvard scientists reported on over 43,000 men, again from the Health Professionals study, and over 71,000 women from the Nurses' Health Study. This time the risk of stroke was assessed and evaluated in terms of lifestyle habits in persons with no history of stroke. If you want to avoid approximately 50% of strokes, you would need to match the following healthy lifestyle habits: no smoking, a body mass index of under 25, 30 minutes a day of moderate activity, modest alcohol intake and a diet in the top 40% of healthy factors (eat your damn vegetables, again and again and again).

Bottom Line: Strokes are devastating, career-ending and often fatal. Cut your risk in half by following lifestyle recommendations derived from over 100,000 persons.

2013

In the MORGEN study, researchers in the Netherlands studied almost 18,000 men and women without heart disease. They followed them for up to 14 years, and in that time more than 600 of the group had heart attacks including deaths. They found that if people followed four steps they were able to lower their risk of heart attacks by 67%:

1. averaging 30 minutes a day of physical activity

2. eating a healthy diet in the Mediterranean style rich in fruits, vegetables and whole grains

3. not smoking

4. enjoying more than one alcoholic beverage a month

People who added a fifth health habit -- sleeping seven or more hours at night on average -- lowered their risk of heart attacks by 83% compared to those not following these steps.

Bottom Line: In addition to the prior health recommendations, you need to sleep! Sleep lets your body recover from a tough day at the office, gym or in the car on the cellphone. Do not cut sleep out of your health plan. If you are not sleeping, see a specialist and find out if you have sleep apnea, which can be tested for at home in your own bed.

2014

The Karolinska Study in Sweden examined more than 20,000 men free of heart issues and followed them for 11 years. They found that there were certain habits that lowered the risk of heart attacks, including:

1. a diet rich in fruits, vegetables, legumes, nuts, whole grains and reduced fat

2. not smoking

3. moderate alcohol consumption daily

4. thin waistlines

5. more than 40 minutes of daily physical activity

Sound familiar? Men who followed all five of these lifestyle habits had an 86% lower chance of developing or dying of heart attacks than those who followed none. Sadly, only 1% of the Swedes studied followed all five habits!

Bottom Line: Be one of the 1%, the group which does all five healthy heart habits. Be at the top of your class in health habits and go almost 90% heart attack-free with little effort and expense. Seriously, how hard is it?

2014

The Caerphilly study in Wales in the UK followed 2,235 men for an amazing 30 years. Five behaviors were tracked for the development of disease and they will sound familiar by now:

1. no smoking

2. normal BMI (under 25)

3. more than three servings daily of fruits and vegetables

4. walking more than two miles daily

5. controlled daily alcohol intake

Men in this study who followed four or five of these habits delayed the development of vascular disease by 12 years, although only 0.1% actually practiced all five! Furthermore, dementia was nearly 70% lower in those following these habits.

Bottom Line: It should be clear by now that if you will make it a habit and promise to follow less than 10 lifestyle habits daily, you will NOT need a cardiologist, a cardiac surgeon, a stroke or cardiac rehab team... or a funeral director, anytime soon.

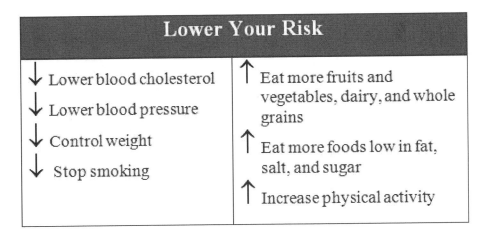

Figure 17. Some strategies to prevent heart attacks

"Bulletproof Your Heart" Summary

Let's summarize what you need to do to prevent a heart by simple daily practices that can make you heart attack-proof:

1. Don't smoke

2. Exercise at least 30 minutes daily, with walking as a baseline habit

3. Keep a trim waist and body weight

4. Eat lots of fruits and vegetables daily with every meal and snack

5. Sleep at night

6. If not an issue, enjoy alcohol up to one modest drink daily for women and two or men (due to differences in alcohol metabolism)

7. I would add a small handful of raw nuts and seeds (particularly flax and chia)

ACTION STEP

You may be managing a company with higher demands on business performance than you demand in your own health life. Go Six Sigma in your lifestyle - or, if you read the list above over and over, go Seven Sigma! Do more than others now to get more than others later, like a heart attack-free career and retirement. No excuses, no whining, just DO

IT! It is easy and powerful to Prevent Not Stent™.

Make sure you take advantage of the bonus techniques that will help

reduce day-to-day stress and can be implemented just about anywhere,

by logging onto

Visit www.drjoelkahn.com/deadexecs OR

Text **PREVENT** to 58885 OR

You can text your email address to 248-731-5145

On the website, you will find a video series that will walk you through

stress management and breathing techniques you can easily implement

into your busy schedule. You'll also find a PDF file to bring with you to

your scheduled doctor appointment entitled, "Questions to Ask Your

Doctor".

Chapter 10

One-Hour Artery Cleaning Is Real

> *"There are a lot of things that go into creating success. I don't like to do just the things I like to do."*
>
> **Michael Dell, CEO of Dell Computer**

Phil was a serious man when he called to meet me, not for an appointment, but to discuss heart disease reversal. He had heard that I was an advocate of nutrition for heart disease management and he wanted to discuss this. We agreed to meet at my house, since he made it clear that he was not shopping for a new cardiologist, but wanted to propose a venture. Perhaps I am too open to ideas, but a few nights later he was seated at my kitchen table drinking tea and telling me his story. He had allowed himself to gain weight and lose focus on his health while he grew his cellular communication business. As he reached his mid 50s, he was finding that playing tennis was getting harder. He initially attributed it to age; but as it progressed, he discussed it with his internist and had a treadmill stress test which he flunked, even though he never felt chest tightness (otherwise known as angina). A heart catheterization followed, performed by another cardiologist, showing advanced heart blockages. After some research, he took himself down to the Cleveland Clinic three hours away from Detroit, planning a bypass. While there, his cardiologist mentioned that a physician on staff did offer a program of preventive measures to reverse heart disease, although he himself really didn't believe they worked. Reverse heart disease? Is that possible? Phil wanted to know, so he met with Dr. Esselstyn and cancelled his heart operation. At my kitchen table, he described how he had changed his diet, had lost 40 pounds, had dropped his cholesterol by nearly 100 points and could again play tennis without limitation. In fact, he had passed a stress test recently that had been abnormal only nine months earlier. His venture? To form a support group for other people looking for the same option. I agreed... and we have never looked back. Although I anticipated gathering 20 people to meet once a quarter, we know have over 500 patients in the group, we meet on at least a monthly basis and many have experienced remarkable improvements in their health with an educated control of their fork and knife. To learn more, visit www.pbnsg.org.

Years ago I saw a sign for a local cleaning service which claimed they offered one-hour artery cleaning and I think they meant shirts and dresses. How about heart arteries? Is this possible? Let's consider where you are at so far.

If you are following the action steps chapter by chapter, you are almost done with your journey of heart attack risk exploration. You may know that both your heart calcium score is zero and your CIMT (Carotid Intima-Media Thickness) is normal for your age. In this case, adapt and follow all the steps in Chapter 7 and you will likely survive your career in great shape and enter retirement years with lots of time left to enjoy. However, the odds are about 60% that you have either had an abnormal coronary calcium CT or CIMT which documents vessel damage or lab values which indicate specific risk targets. What then? What if your calcium score is greater than zero, or your CIMT demonstrates a vascular age greater than your driver's license, or your lab values say you are aging too fast? Is it all futile and your path is pre-set and likely to be riddled by medical illness?

"No way!" is the strong answer! There are ample studies demonstrating that even if you have cardiovascular disease right now, even if you have had a stent, bypass surgery, heart attack or other documented advanced disease, SO much can be done - including the possibility of reversing your heart disease and regaining a youthful constitution. This is even more accessible if you have been found to have silent heart disease by CT or CIMT, since you are probably at an earlier stage of disease. Let's explore how that can be achieved. I will paint the broad strokes; if you want all the details, just come see me and I will teach you the finer points.

1. **First, the cold, hard truth**. You might have serious silent

heart disease. If your coronary artery calcium CT scan came back abnormal, you may need a stress test. This is definitely the case if the score was high, certainly over 400 and possible even at a lower level of abnormality based on where the calcium is located (the left main [LM] and left anterior descending [LAD] arteries supply the most blood to the heart and are the most important if heavily calcified). That is what the American College of Cardiology recommends. Yes, I discussed limitations in stress testing previously; but if you have a lot of silent heart artery disease you need to be sure that you can exercise on a treadmill or take a chemical infusion stress test without showing reduced blood flow. An abnormal stress test after a high coronary artery calcium CT scan would suggest that you have an advanced heart artery narrowing which may need further evaluation with regards to lifestyle, medication and possibly heart catheterization. Some individuals simply will never feel angina pain, shortness of breath or other clinical warning signs and the first evidence that the calcification was ominous could be a massive heart attack or death. Make sure you are NOT one of them.

2.   **Diet reverses heart disease**. Have you ever heard that before? That you could have an 80% blocked heart or brain artery and that you could turn the clock back and reduce the blockage by changing the way you eat? It is true. My friend David Katz, MD, Professor of Medicine at Yale University and head of Preventive Medicine there, often says "your fork will determine your fate" and it is never more true than in heart disease reversal. There are several different lines of evidence which support this bold statement as a proven scientific fact and they are summarized here.

The Ornish Lifestyle Heart Diet

Dr. Dean Ornish offered one of the first clues that heart disease could be reversed by diet by using advanced medical techniques to prove the point. He was training in cardiology in San Francisco in the 1980s when he organized a trial offering nutrition and lifestyle management to patients with documented severe heart blockages. His program, The Lifestyle Heart Trial, was published in 1990 with data after one year and in 1998 with data for five years of follow-up. His research protocol offered patients with advanced heart disease a vegetarian diet with low fat (about 10% total fat calories), moderate exercise with an emphasis on walking, stress management with meditation and breathing practices, smoking cessation and group support. Patients had sophisticated angiograms and stress tests before changing their diets and in follow-up. Heart blockages showed reversal on follow-up angiography at one and five years much more commonly than when compared to a control group whose blockages worsened during the study period. The number of heart attacks was cut in half in the treatment group which ate mainly plants. Patients reported feeling better, having less chest pain and having better sexual function. Dr. Ornish later expanded his treatment group to over 2,000 patients, as reported in the medical literature, and gained approval in 2010 to have Medicare pay for this therapy in an approved center. Heart disease is reversible - if you will change your lifestyle to do Ornish, not Cornish.

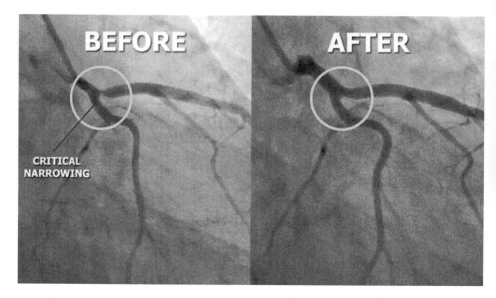

Figure 18. A coronary angiogram showing a narrowing before and near complete resolution after a reversal diet

The Esselstyn Diet

Doctor Caldwell Esselstyn was an esteemed breast surgeon at the Cleveland Clinic when he became interested in heart disease. He shared a locker with the first surgeon in the world who had performed heart bypass surgery and began reading about why heart disease develops. He found societies with little or no heart attacks and studied their lifestyle. He became convinced that heart disease could be prevented or reversed with changes in nutrition. He began treating patients at the Clinic who were not eligible for bypass surgery or angioplasty. They often had advanced heart issues and a very poor prognosis. He showed them how to eat a completely plant-based diet with less than 10% fat, often referred to as the "Essy" diet. He met with them regularly to provide group support beginning in 1985 and his dedicated wife Anne showed them how to prepare delicious meals. The subjects reported feeling much better within weeks, often walking further, taking less heart medication and needing hospital care far less than before the Essy diet. Several had before and after heart angiograms and stress tests and remarkable reversal of blocked arteries was documented. In a follow-up period of more than 12 years, he documented the absence of heart events in treated patients, as well as an improvement in vitality and sexual function. In the summer of 2014, he updated his results to a much larger group of subjects and the same amazing improvements held true after all these years. His book Prevent and Reverse Heart Disease, published in 2007, has even longer positive follow-up data. I have had the pleasure of knowing Dr. Esselstyn for many years and have traveled to the Cleveland Clinic to study with him. Now in his 80s, he is still focused on stopping heart disease, witnessing the very

last heart attack and enriching the lives of as many persons as possible.

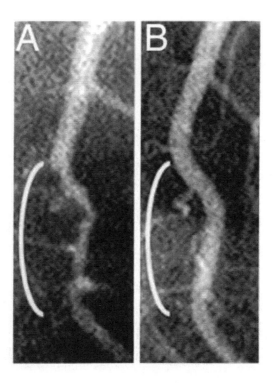

Figure 19. An angiogram showing severe narrowing on the left and reversed on the right after dietary therapy

The Lyon Diet Heart Study

This groundbreaking scientific trial reported in the 1990s studied

over 400 patients with a prior heart attack. The diet featured a

Mediterranean-style menu, including more bread, vegetables, fish, fruit and less red meat and fat. If oil was used, canola oil was the preferred choice and wine was permitted. The diet was about 30% fat so it differed from the program of Drs. Ornish and Esselstyn. The study was stopped early because the group eating more vegetables and less meat and animal fat experienced far fewer repeat heart attacks. In fact, the patients following the Lyon diet had a 50% to 70% lower chance of recurrent heart disease such as heart attacks, death and hospitalizations during a follow-up period of more than four years. The subjects studied did not have angiography before and after, so we cannot say for sure that heart lesions improved during the study period; I also believe that the fat content in the diet was too high for a long-term strategy.

Chelation Therapy

Chelation therapy is a treatment which has been available for decades. The word chelation comes from the Latin word for "claw," with the idea that bad factors in the body can be grabbed and removed. Chelation therapy was developed to treat environmental exposure to heavy metal toxicity, such as an acute burden of exposure to lead at work in a foundry. While using it, some practitioners noted improvements in symptoms of heart disease in the patients they were treating, and chelation began to be used in some clinics for heart patients. (There's quite a large body of science which suggests that "heavy metal" toxins like lead, mercury, cadmium and arsenic can poison systems important to heart health, so even at that time, it made sense.)

Physicians in traditional practices, however, viewed chelation therapy as quackery, since there was only minimal science to support it. As a physician, I advised my patients to avoid it, since I couldn't find much research to support its use.

Fast forward to the past few years. Over a decade ago, the National Institute of Health agreed to provide $31 million to fund the "definitive trial" for chelation therapy. This trial was called the TACT trial (Trial to Assess Chelation Therapy).

Over the course of about 10 years, more than 1,700 people who had suffered a heart attack received real chelation therapy or sham IV therapies, planned once a week for 40 sessions. Despite the fact that not all patients finished the treatments, and that enrollment was slow, the trial was completed and the results were presented for the first time in November 2012.

These results showed that chelation therapy modestly reduced the risk of bad cardiovascular outcomes. Although the study provided a platform for further research, researchers cautioned that on its own it wasn't conclusive enough to support routine use of the therapy after heart attack. However, since the data on the TACT trial was originally released, a number of additional papers have been published. Taken together, this body of research has identified that:

- Overall, chelation therapy modestly reduced bad outcomes (hospitalization for chest pain, stroke, heart attack and need for a stent) compared to the placebo group.

- In patients with a prior heart attack and diabetes, chelation therapy reduced bad outcomes during five years of follow-up by nearly 40%. Powerful therapy!

- In patients with a large heart attack before chelation therapy, the treatment also reduced bad outcomes in follow-up by nearly 40%.

- When chelation therapy was combined with a high dose of oral multivitamins, even more benefit was obtained with chelation therapy.

- Adverse effects from chelation therapy were infrequent.

Imagine a new pill which reduced the risk of heart problems by 40% in large numbers of patients. Do you think it would generate billions of dollars in sales? By contrast, since the TACT trial published its results, the therapy has made no impact on the routine care of patients and there is no reimbursement for the treatments (cash payments only).

There are some challenges to the therapy: IV chelation therapy is more involved than taking a pill (there are oral agents which can be used but these weren't studied in the TACT trial) and chelation therapy is not covered by insurance programs.

In my practice I have identified physicians in my area who have trained in chelation therapy and have experience with heavy metal testing and treatment. I've referred patients to these colleagues to discuss a course of oral or IV chelation therapy. Oral agents that create a chelating effect are available from reliable supplement companies and I have used these in patient-programs. I have also routinely prescribed oral agents like n-acetyl cysteine (NAC), organic cruciferous vegetables (broccoli sprouts, cauliflower, greens and bok choy) and leafy green vegetables to promote the detoxification of chemicals from the body. Broccoli sprouts added to the diet have been demonstrated to speed the elimination of toxins in air pollution from the body. Avoiding exposures to heavy metals by not smoking, limiting fish consumption, being aware of air and water contamination and considering the removal of dental fillings made with mercury is also important.

3.   **Medications and supplements.**

So far, the magic cure-all that comes in a prescription or vitamin bottle is elusive. However, if silent early heart disease has been found on your tests, there are some considerations. You surely have heard the word "statins"; these are prescription cholesterol-lowering medications like

Lipitor and Crestor which are widely prescribed. Can they reverse heart artery blockages like those found on coronary artery calcium CT scans? Several human studies have looked at the progression of coronary artery calcification over time, as to whether statins can slow or reverse the inevitable worsening year after year. In fact, the degree of coronary calcification usually worsens by 20-30% yearly. These studies have shown that lowering the cholesterol level can slow the worsening of heart artery calcification. At least one study, using the statin Baycol (which is no longer available due to a high side-effect profile), actually lowered the measures of coronary calcium. If you are taking a statin medication, protect yourself by taking 200 mg of CoQ10 daily to prevent depletion of this crucial energy co-factor. In some patients, I extend mitochondrial support (the powerhouse of all cells) to several additional agents to prevent statin-induced muscle pain or fatigue.

Are there other pills, beyond statin prescription medications, which might speed heart disease reversal? Small studies have indicated that concentrated supplement of fruits and vegetables, aged garlic tablets, omega-3 fatty acids (as can be found in fish oil capsules or flax and chia seeds and walnuts) and Vitamin K supplements may all slow or possibly reverse calcified arteries. In my clinic I use all of these modalities.

4.   Sauna: Sweat the Small and the Big Stuff Away

While most of us assume that sweating during a workout or in a sauna may be good for us, my hunch is that most of us don't know why. The fact is, sweating is one of the best ways to remove toxins from our body and medical research can actually explain how this happens. We live in a world where industrial toxins have become so prevalent that none of us are free from exposure. In fact, the umbilical cord of a newborn baby can be sampled and will reveal an average of over 200 synthetic chemicals, some of them with carcinogenic potential.

Heavy metals such as mercury, lead, cadmium and arsenic are abundant in our environment and endocrine disruptors such as phthalates and bisphenol A can be found in our blood and urine. What does the science say about removing these risks to our health through our sweat pores?

Sweating can help eliminate phthalates.

Phthalates are used in plastic toys, cooking utensils, fragrances, nail polish, cosmetics and paints. Researchers in Canada examined blood, urine and sweat concentrations of various phthalates. They found that the concentration of these chemicals was twice as high in sweat as in urine and suggested that perspiration may help eliminate some toxic compounds.

Sweating can help eliminate BPA.

Bisphehol A (BPA) is widely used to make clear plastics, but is also used in cash register receipts, water pipes, electronics and eyeglass lenses. This compound has been known for years to have estrogenic properties and exposure to it has been linked to obesity, early puberty, sexual dysfunction and miscarriage. The same group of Canadian researchers found BPA in the sweat of 80% of subjects tested. Some of these people had no detectable levels in their blood or urine, which suggests that sweat was the best way to excrete stored bisphenol A.

Sweating can help eliminate heavy metals.

153

The heavy metals arsenic, cadmium, lead and mercury are confirmed or suspected carcinogens and are toxic in all sorts of ways to your body. They are known to harm the heart, brain, kidney and immunological systems. Heavy metals are present in water, food, dental amalgams, cigarettes and industrial emissions. Studies show sweat can concentrate arsenic up to 10 times more than blood, cadmium up to 25 times more than blood, lead up to 300 times more than blood, and mercury somewhat more than blood, leading to effective elimination.

So how does this relate to you? Sweating has been considered a therapy since the Roman baths, Aboriginal sweat lodges, Scandinavian saunas and Turkish baths of yesteryear. Recently, infrared saunas have become available; these are cooler than other saunas but penetrate the skin deeper to promote sweating and toxin excretion. Can infrared saunas heal your silent heart disease?

Infrared Sauna to Heal Artery Disease

Doctors in Japan have been working for over 20 years testing the benefits of infrared dry sauna therapy in some of the sickest heart and vascular patients, and they've published nearly 20 research articles showing this as a major breakthrough. They've used a technique called waon therapy, from the Japanese words wa for soothing and on for warmth, or so-called soothing warmth therapy. Here's how it works: patients sit in an infrared sauna set at 60° C (140° F) for 15 minutes, followed by resting outside the sauna for 30 minutes, wrapped in towels. People are encouraged to drink water to compensate for the perspiration. And what can waon therapy do for the general health of heart patients?

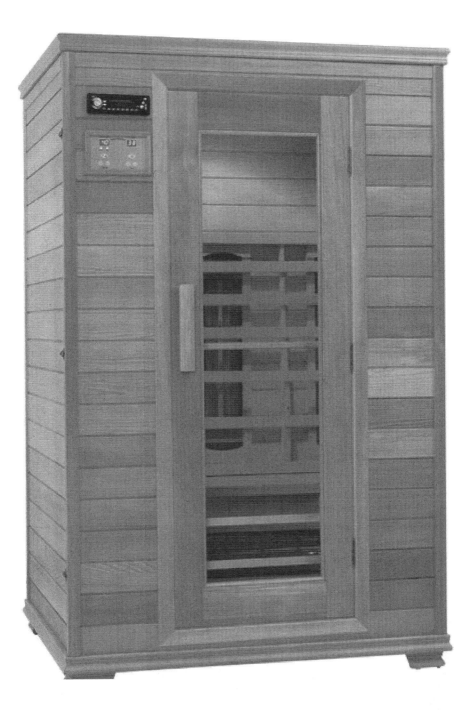

Figure 20. An infrared sauna suitable for home or office

Waon therapy improves the health of arteries.

The lining of your arteries is a single layer called your endothelium. Acting much more than a simple barrier for blood cells, these cells produce dozens of compounds which cause arteries to resist developing plaque, blood clots or constriction. Waon therapy has been shown to improve the function of these cells and the blood flow they carry.

Waon therapy lowers the "fire" in your body

Whether you have a disease, eat junk and processed food, are stressed or are overweight, your blood is filled every day with molecules triggering inflammation and destructive processes. When measured after a few weeks of waon therapy, the levels of these molecules decrease, both in patients with heart disease and just the "average Joe" living the stressed Western lifestyle.

Waon therapy improves exercise ability

A hallmark of heart disease is the reduced ability to exercise.

Perhaps due to a healthier endothelium and less inflammation, after treatments with waon therapy people demonstrate a greater ability to walk, regardless of whether they were normally limited by heart or leg vascular issues.

Waon therapy may save lives

In an amazing study of 129 patients with bad heart problems, patients treated with waon therapy at least two times a week were compared to similar patients who did not get the soothing warmth therapy. Over five years of follow-up, the rate of rehospitalization and death was half in the waon-treated patients compared to the others! If a drug reduced hospitalization and death by 50% in these patients, it would easily be a billion-dollar winner.

"Bulletproof Your Heart" Summary

1. Scientific studies over 25 years show that diet can reverse heart disease

2. Chelation has the potential to reduce heart events and eliminate toxins

3. Sweating, particularly in an infrared sauna, is a proven therapy

4. A clean diet, exercise and stress management are always the foundation

ACTION STEPS

I would strongly encourage you to consider a home infrared sauna unit. I have a one in my bedroom.

Furthermore, you can take advantage of bonus techniques which will

help reduce day-to-day stress and can be implemented just about

anywhere, by logging onto

Visit www.drjoelkahn.com/deadexecs OR

Text **PREVENT** to 58885 OR

You can text your email address to 248-731-5145

On the website, you will find a video series that will walk you through

stress management and breathing techniques you can easily implement

into your busy schedule. You'll also find a PDF file to bring with you to

your scheduled doctor appointment entitled, "Questions to Ask Your

Doctor".

Chapter 11

Conclusion

"Balance suggests a perfect equilibrium. There is no such thing. That is a false expectation... There are going to be priorities and dimensions of your life; how you integrate them is how you find true happiness."

Denise Morrison, CEO of Campbell Soup

If you have made it this far, I am excited that you have learned the habits and skills to live a long and productive life free of the tragedy of a heart attack. Although I do not want to offend anyone, I view heart attacks as mistakes, missed opportunities and almost CARE-less events that can maim or kill great people in the prime of their lives. A few years back, PBS featured an interview with President Bill Clinton called The Last

Heart Attack. In it, President Clinton shared how after his open heart surgery, he assumed he would have a clean bill of health for a long time. When, only a few years later, he was back with more symptoms and a documented loss of one of his bypass grafts, he decided to change his lifestyle dramatically and strive for freedom from future heart disease and attacks. He outlined the steps he took to alter his diet and exercise programs to reach this goal (although I am concerned that recent reports indicate he may be wavering from his commitment).

Just like President Clinton, I look forward to the Last Heart Attack. We do not need to read about any more tragedies like Imre Molnar or any other of the business heroes who lives have been cut short by heart disease. I know we can reach that goal for over 90% of readers, and with the complete program outlined here, I think 100% protection is not out of reach. A bulletproof heart is not a fantasy. No matter what barriers you have to overcome in adopting the complete heart attack prevention program I have outlined, the objections can be surmounted with a dream, a drive and a plan to learn new skills and habits. I often say to my patients that a person with good health has 1,000 dreams - while a person with poor health has only one dream. For the sake of your business plans, perhaps your shareholders, certainly for your children and family and your spouse - but mainly for your own survival - make no excuses; execute a business plan to recapture your health and live a heart attack-free life.

You can take advantage of bonus techniques which will help reduce

day-to-day stress and can be implemented just about anywhere, by

logging onto

Visit www.drjoelkahn.com/deadexecs OR

Text **PREVENT** to 58885 OR

You can text your email address to 248-731-5145

On the website, you will find a video series that will walk you through

stress management and breathing techniques you can easily implement

into your busy schedule. You'll also find a PDF file to bring with you to

your scheduled doctor appointment entitled, "Questions to Ask Your

Doctor".

Made in the USA
Middletown, DE
30 December 2015